ULCERATIVE COLITIS COOKBOOK

MEGA BUNDLE – 4 Manuscripts in 1 – 160+ Ulcerative Colitis - friendly recipes including casseroles, stew, side dishes, and pasta for a delicious and tasty diet

TABLE OF CONTENTS

ROAST RECIPES 10

ROASTED SQUASH...10

ROASTED CUCUMBER 11

SOUP RECIPES 12

ZUCCHINI SOUP..12

BEAN SOUP 13

SIDE DISHES 15

RICE PAPER ROLLS 15

CHICKEN NOODLE SALAD 17

SHREDDED SWEET POTATO HASH BROWNS.........................19

SPAGHETTI WITH MEATBALLS..20

HOMEMADE CHICKEN NUGGETS 21

GRILLED VEGETABLES...22

PORK KEBABS 23

TUNA PASTA SALAD 25

ROASTED CHICKPEAS 26

GRAIN FREE FAJITAS...27

FISH TACOS...29

AVOCADO SANDWICH...31

GREEN PESTO PASTA..32

CAULIFLOWER STEAKS WITH LEMON SAUCE 33

KUNG PAO CAULIFLOWER..35

RICE, KALE AND AVOCADO BOWL...37

CHICKEN MEATBALLS AND CAULIFLOWER RICE....................39

PINEAPPLE CHICKEN AND LETTUCE WRAPS.........................41

ROASTED SALMON WITH POTATOES 42

GUT ENERGY BOOSTING BOWL 43

BALED EGGS WITH ZOODLES..44

CHICKEN WITH BAKED VEGGIES...45

VEGGIE STIR-FRY 46

WALDORF SALAD 47

CRANBERRY SALAD 48

ARUGULA SALAD 49

MANDARIN SALAD 50

BEAN FAJITAS 52

TOFU SALAD...53

PAD THAI SALAD..54

STEW RECIPES 55

BEEF STEW 55

IRISH STEW..57

CASSEROLE RECIPES..58

CHICKEN CASSEROLE...58

RICE CASSEROLE 60

PIZZA RECIPES 61

MUSHROOM PIZZA 61

CASSEROLE PIZZA 63

SECOND COOKBOOK...64

SOUP RECIPES 65

CAULIFLOWER SOUP 65

GARLIC SOUP...66

LEEK SOUP...67

CARROT SOUP 68

CELERY SOUP...69

SIDE DISHES 70

GREEN PESTO PASTA...70

FIESTA SHRIMP 71

DIJON VINAIGRETTE 72

COTTAGE CHEESE CASSEROLE..73

FRENCH DRESSING 74

TAPENADE 75

MUSHROOM BACON...76

ZUCCHINI CASSEROLE 77

NOODLES WITH PARMESAN CHEESE 78

BALSAMIC CHICKEN 79

STEAMED SALMON 80

ROASTED POTATOES 81

FRESH SALAD...82

CHICKEN SALAD..83

CRANBERRY PECAN SALAD...85

PEAR SALAD...86

WATERMELON SALAD 87

POTATO SALAD 88

SOUTHWESTERN SALAD..89

TOMATO SALAD 90

MELON SALAD..91

RED CABBAGE FRITATTA 92

KALE FRITATTA 93

BRUSSEL SPROUTS FRITATTA 94

BROCCOLI FRITATTA..95

SPAGHETI SQUASH..96

SPICY MUSSELS...97

SHRIMP FAJITAS 98

GARLIC CLAMS 99

CROCKPOT CHICKEN..100

ROASTED SQUASH..101

CUCUMBER CHIPS..102

SQUASH CHIPS..103

PIZZA 104

ZUCCHINI PIZZA..104

CHICKEN PIZZA..105

CIABATTA PIZZA 106

SHRIMP PIZZA..107

THIRD COOKBOOK..108

BREAKFAST RECIPES 109

FRENCH TOAST..109

BREAKFAST QUINOA 110

CHEESE SANDWICH 111

MORNING POT 112

BREAKFAST ROLL-UPS 113

BANANA BREAD 115

BLUEBERRY PANCAKES..117

NUTS AND DATES BARS..119

APPLE PORRIDGE..120

MORNING GRANOLA..121

BLUEBERRY FRENCH TOAST 123

PUMPKIN MUFFINS..124

MORNING YOGURT 125

CRANBERRY WALNUT SCONES..126

PIZZA MUFFINS 127

CINNAMON CAKE 128

ORANGE SCONES..130

CREPES 131

MINI BAGELS 132

PUMPKING CRANBERRY GRANOLA 133

ORANGE BISCUITS 135

BAGELS 136

LEMON MUFFINS 137

BREAKFAST BARS...138

MORNING SCONES...139

PUMPKIN MUFFINS..140

PALEO PORRIDGE 141

TART RECIPES..142

STRAWBERRY TART 142

HAZELNUT TART 143

PIE RECIPES 144

PEACH PECAN PIE...144

OREO PIE 145

GRAPEFRUIT PIE 146

SMOOTHIE RECIPES 147

TURMERIC-MANGO SMOOTHIE..147

AVOCADO-KALE SMOOTHIE..148

BUTTERMILK SMOOTHIE 149

GREEN SMOOTHIE..150

FRUIT SMOOTHIE 151

MANGO SMOOTHIE 152

DREAMSICLE SMOOTHIE 153

ICE-CREAM RECIPES 154

RICOTTA ICE-CREAM 154

SAFFRON ICE-CREAM 155

FOURTH COOKBOOK 156

SIDE DISHES 157

CAULIFLOWER STEAKS WITH LEMON SAUCE 157

KUNG PAO CAULIFLOWER 159

RICE, KALE AND AVOCADO BOWL 161

CHICKEN MEATBALLS AND CAULIFLOWER RICE 163

PINEAPPLE CHICKEN AND LETTUCE WRAPS 165

ROASTED SALMON WITH POTATOES 166

GUT ENERGY BOOSTING BOWL 167

BALED EGGS WITH ZOODLES 168

CHICKEN WITH BAKED VEGGIES 169

VEGGIE STIR-FRY 170

GREEK PIZZA 171

CHICKEN PIZZA 172

FIESTA SHRIMP 173

CAULIFLOWER FRITTERS 174

FRENCH TOAST SANDWICHES 176

GREEK MIXED VEGETABLES 177

GRILLED SALMON STEAKS 179

ORIENTAL GREENS 180

BROCCOLI CASSEROLE 181

RED ONION FRITATTA 182

SPINACH FRITATTA 183

CHEESE FRITATTA 184

RHUBARB FRITATTA 185

BROCCOLI FRITATTA 186

TOMATO RISOTTO 187

SQUASH QUICHE 188

TOMATO TARTS...189

TOMATO AND ONION PASTA...190

ROASTED SQUASH...191

BRUSSELS SPROUT CHIPS 192

PASTA...193

SIMPLE SPAGHETTI..193

SHRIMP PASTA 195

PASTA WITH OLIVES AND TOMATOES 196

SALAD...197

TOMATO AND CUCUMBER SALAD 197

RADICCHIO AND TOMATO SALAD 198

BROCCOLI SALAD WITH CRANBERRIES...199

SMOKED SALMON SALAD 200

SHRIMP AND EGGS SALAD 201

AVOCADO SALAD 202

CHICKEN SALAD WITH PINE NUTS..203

APPLE SALAD 205

BEET AND CARROT SALAD..206

equally by a Committee of the American Bar Association and a Committee of Publishers and Associations.

Introduction

Ulcerative Colitis recipes for personal enjoyment but also for family enjoyment. You will love them for sure for how easy it is to prepare them.

ROASTED SQUASH

Serves: **3-4**
Prep Time: **10**   Minutes

Cook Time: **20**   Minutes

Total Time: **30**   Minutes

INGREDIENTS

- 2 delicata squashes
- 2 tablespoons olive oil
- 1 tsp curry powder
- 1 tsp salt

DIRECTIONS

1. Preheat the oven to 400 F
2. Cut everything in half lengthwise
3. Toss everything with olive oil and place onto a prepared baking sheet
4. Roast for 18-20 minutes at 400 F or until golden brown
5. When ready remove from the oven and serve

ROASTED CUCUMBER

Serves: **3-4**
Prep Time: **10**   Minutes

Cook Time: **20**   Minutes

Total Time: **30**   Minutes

INGREDIENTS

- 2 lb. cucumber
- 2 tablespoons olive oil
- 1 tsp curry powder
- 1 tsp salt

DIRECTIONS

1. Preheat the oven to 400 F
2. Cut everything in half lengthwise
3. Toss everything with olive oil and place onto a prepared baking sheet
4. Roast for 18-20 minutes at 400 F or until golden brown
5. When ready remove from the oven and serve

SOUP RECIPES

ZUCCHINI SOUP

Serves: **4**

Prep Time: **10**   Minutes

Cook Time: **20**   Minutes

Total Time: **30**   Minutes

INGREDIENTS

- 1 tablespoon olive oil
- 1 lb. zucchini
- ¼ red onion
- ½ cup all-purpose flour
- ¼ tsp salt
- ¼ tsp pepper
- 1 can vegetable broth
- 1 cup heavy cream

DIRECTIONS

1. In a saucepan heat olive oil and sauté zucchini until tender
2. Add remaining ingredients to the saucepan and bring to a boil
3. When all the vegetables are tender transfer to a blender and blend until smooth
4. Pour soup into bowls, garnish with parsley and serve

BEAN SOUP

Serves: **4**
Prep Time: **10**   Minutes

Cook Time: **230**   Minutes

Total Time: **240**   Minutes

INGREDIENTS

- 2 cups beans
- 1/2 tsp salt
- 2 cups chicken broth
- 7 cups water
- 2 tsp sauce
- ½ 10-ounce package onions
- 2 clove garlic
- 3 bay leaves
- ½ tsp dried rosemary
- 1 tsp dried sage
- 2 tsp dried thyme

DIRECTIONS

1. Place the bean mixture in a pot with the rest of ingredients
2. Cook over medium heat until the soup boils
3. Reduce the heat and simmer for 3-4 hours

4. **When ready remove from heat and serve**

SIDE DISHES

RICE PAPER ROLLS

Serves: **4**

Prep Time: **10**   Minutes

Cook Time: **15**   Minutes

Total Time: **25**   Minutes

INGREDIENTS

- 1 cucumber
- 1 red capsicum
- 1 carrot
- 1 avocado
- 2 oz. pea sprouts
- ¾ coriander
- ¾ cup mint
- 2 oz. peanuts
- 2 tablespoons chili sauce
- 1 tablespoon soy sauce
- 2 tablespoons lime juice

DIRECTIONS

1. Place all the vegetables on a plate
2. In a bowl mix chili sauce, lime juice and soy sauce

3. Some one rice paper roll in a bowl of water and then place vegetables on the wrapper
4. Fold up the bottom of the wrapped, and roll u to enclose filling
5. Place on a tray, serve with dipping sauce

CHICKEN NOODLE SALAD

Serves: **4**

Prep Time: **10**   Minutes

Cook Time: **30**   Minutes

Total Time: **40**   Minutes

INGREDIENTS

- 1 lb. tenderloins
- 2 oz. rice noodle
- 1 carrot
- 1 celery stalk
- 1 cucumber
- ¼ capsicum
- 1 tablespoon peanuts

DRESSING

- 1 onion
- 1 garlic clove
- ½ cup soy sauce
- ½ cup rice vinegar
- 1 tsp sugar
- 1 tsp sesame oil

DIRECTIONS

1. Place all dressing ingredients in a jar and mix well
2. In a bowl place all salad ingredients and mix well
3. Pour dressing over salad and serve

SHREDDED SWEET POTATO HASH BROWNS

Serves: 2
Prep Time: 10   minutes
Cook Time: 30   minutes
Total Time: 40   minutes

INGREDIENTS

- 7 oz. sweet potatoes
- 3 tablespoons butter
- 1 tablespoon dried sage
- 1/8 tablespoon black pepper
- 1/8 tablespoon salt

DIRECTIONS

1. Shred the potatoes and place them in a strainer.
2. Use a rubber spatula and press the excess water.
3. Place the potatoes on a paper towel and pat as dry as possible.
4. Put the potatoes in a bowl and add sage, salt and pepper.
5. Place the butter in a skillet over high heat.
6. When the butter is melted add the potatoes.
7. Toss well for 5 minutes and gather them together into two piles.
8. Cook the potatoes slowly.
9. Cook on each side for 3 minutes.

SPAGHETTI WITH MEATBALLS

Serves: **2**

Prep Time: **10**   minutes

Cook Time: **35**   minutes

Total Time: **45**   minutes

INGREDIENTS

- 4 quarts' water
- 5 meatballs
- ½ tomato sauce
- ½ ounces Parmigiano-Reggiano
- 2 ounces' spaghetti noodles

DIRECTIONS

1. In a large pot add water to high heat
2. Add spaghetti noodles
3. Add the meatballs and tomato sauce in a medium sauce pan while the pasta is cooking
4. Remove the noodles and allow them to drain
5. Place the noodles in the sauce with the meatballs

Serves: **4**

Prep Time: **10** Minutes

Cook Time: **30** Minutes

Total Time: **40** Minutes

INGREDIENTS

- 1 lbs. chicken breast
- 2 small eggs
- ¼ tsp garlic powder
- ¼ tsp salt
- ¼ cup breadcrumbs
- 1 ½ cups cauliflower

DIRECTIONS

1. Preheat oven to 325 F and place a baking tray in
2. In a bowl mix garlic powder, salt and egg and whisk together
3. In another bowl mix cauliflower and breadcrumbs, dip the chicken into the mixture
4. Bake for 20-25 minutes on each side

GRILLED VEGETABLES

Serves: **4**
Prep Time: **10**   Minutes

Cook Time: **10**   Minutes

Total Time: **20**   Minutes

INGREDIENTS

- 1 tablespoon olive oil
- ¼ tsp salt
- 2 bell peppers
- 1 bunch asparagus
- 2 small zucchinis
- 1 tablespoon rice vinegar
- 1 tablespoon oregano
- 1 eggplant

DIRECTIONS

1. In a bowl whisk salt, oregano, vinegar and olive oil
2. Place the vegetables into a bowl
3. Place vegetables on a grill
4. Cook eggplant and zucchini pieces for 5-6 minutes per side
5. Toss asparagus and cool for 4-5 minutes
6. Transfer to a plate and serve when ready

PORK KEBABS

Serves: *8*
Prep Time: *10* Minutes

Cook Time: *15* Minutes

Total Time: *25* Minutes

INGREDIENTS

- ½ cup fresh basil
- 22 red globe grapes
- ¼ Tsp allspice
- 1 lb. pork loin chop
- 1 tsp cumin
- ¼ tsp cardamom
- ¼ tsp salt
- 2 tsp fenugreek seeds
- ¼ black pepper

DIRECTIONS

1. In a bowl mix cumin, cardamom, salt, pepper, fenugreek and set aside
2. Cut the pork and sprinkle the mixture onto the pork cubes and stir until well coated
3. For each kebab slide a cube of pork into the skewer and alternate with basil wrapped grapes

4. Preheat the grill and cook for 10-15 minutes

TUNA PASTA SALAD

Serves: **4**

Prep Time: **10**   Minutes

Cook Time: **30**   Minutes

Total Time: **40**   Minutes

INGREDIENTS

- 3 cups bow tie pasta
- 1 cup cherry tomatoes
- 1 tablespoon olive oil
- 2 tablespoons wine vinegar
- 1 tsp mustard
- ¼ cup parsley
- 1 tin tuna

DIRECTIONS

1. Combine all ingredients together and mix well
2. Serve when ready

Serves: *4*

Prep Time: *10*   Minutes

Cook Time: *30*   Minutes

Total Time: *40*   Minutes

INGREDIENTS

- 2 cans chickpeas
- 1 tsp olive oil
- 1 tsp salt
- 1 tsp pepper
- 1 tsp thyme
- 1 tsp rosemary

DIRECTIONS

1. Preheat oven to 350 F
2. Line an oven tray with baking paper, toss chickpeas in salt, pepper and oil
3. Pour mixture over baking paper and roast for 20-25 minutes
4. Remove and serve

Serves: **3**

Prep Time: **10**   Minutes

Cook Time: **10**   Minutes

Total Time: **20**   Minutes

INGREDIENTS

- 1 tablespoon avocado oil
- 3 carrots
- 3 large nori sheets
- 1 tomato
- 1 tablespoon fresh cilantro
- 1 red pepper
- 1 green bell pepper
- 1 while onion
- 1 jalapeno

DIRECTIONS

1. In a skillet sauce avocado oil, onion, jalapeno, white onion, salt and pepper for 6-7 minutes
2. Remove from heat and place mixture in a bowl
3. Sauté carrots with pepper and salt for 5-6 minutes
4. Combine coconut milk with curry powder and combine with red onion, sea s alt and pepper

5. Lay the nori sheets and top with pepper mixture and carrots and drizzle with coconut milk

FISH TACOS

Serves: **4**

Prep Time: **10** Minutes

Cook Time: **30** Minutes

Total Time: **40** Minutes

INGREDIENTS

- 8 fish fingers
- ¼ cabbage
- tacos
- guacamole
- 2 avocados
- salt
- coriander
- juice of 1 lime

Salsa

- 2 cherry tomatoes
- ½ onion
- 1 tablespoon vinegar
- 8 jalapeno slices
- juice 1 lime
- salt

  Spicy mayo
- ½ cup mayo

- 1 tablespoon paprika
- ½ cup ketchup
- juice 1 lime

DIRECTIONS

1. For salsa add all the ingredients into a blender and blend until smooth, place into a bowl and set aside
2. Mash avocado with salt, lime juice and mix with coriander
3. Mix your spicy mayo in a bowl, heat your tacos and pour the mixture on the tacos
4. Serve when ready

AVOCADO SANDWICH

Serves: *1*
Prep Time: *10* Minutes

Cook Time: *10* Minutes

Total Time: *20* Minutes

INGREDIENTS

- 1 avocado
- juice of 1 lemon pinch of salt
- coriander
- 6 rashers of bacon
- 4 slices bread
- 2 eggs
- ¼ tablespoon hot sauce

DIRECTIONS

1. In a pan add bacon and cook over medium heat
2. In a bowl mix lemon juice, salt, avocado and coriander
3. Toss your bread in the pan and crack an egg into the bread (make a hole before)
4. Add the avocado mixture over the bread and top with bacon

Serves: *2*

Prep Time: *5*   Minutes

Cook Time: *15*   Minutes

Total Time: *20*   Minutes

INGREDIENTS

- 4 oz. spaghetti
- 2 cups basil leaves
- 2 garlic cloves
- ¼ cup olive oil
- 2 tablespoons parmesan cheese
- ½ tsp black pepper

DIRECTIONS

1. Bring water to a boil and add pasta
2. In a blend add parmesan cheese, basil leaves, garlic and blend
3. Add olive oil, pepper and blend again
4. Pour pesto onto pasta and serve when ready

CAULIFLOWER STEAKS WITH LEMON SAUCE

Serves: **4**

Prep Time: **10**   Minutes

Cook Time: **10**   Minutes

Total Time: **20**   Minutes

INGREDIENTS

- 1 head cauliflower
- 2 tablespoons olive oil
- 2 tsp paprika

LEMON SAUCE

- 1 cup parsley leaves
- ¼ cup mint leaves
- 1 garlic clove
- ¼ cup olive oil
- ¼ cup green onion
- Juice of 1 lemon

DIRECTIONS

1. In a blender add all ingredients for the lemon sauce and blend until smooth
2. For the cauliflower steak, cut cauliflower into thick slices and rub with olive oil

3. Sprinkle with spices and place the cauliflower in a skillet
4. Cook for 4-5 minutes per side
5. When ready remove and serve with lemon sauce

KUNG PAO CAULIFLOWER

Serves: **4**
Prep Time: **10** Minutes

Cook Time: **30** Minutes

Total Time: **40** Minutes

INGREDIENTS

- 2 tablespoons olive oil
- salt
- 2 scallions
- ¼ cup cilantro
- 1 head cauliflower
- 1 tablespoon sesame seeds

SAUCE

- 1 tablespoon rice wine vinegar
- 1 tablespoon ginger
- 1 tsp olive oil
- 1 tablespoon soy sauce
- 1 tablespoon hoisin sauce

DIRECTIONS

1. In a bowl combine all sauce ingredients together and mix well
2. For the cauliflower heat the olive oil in a skillet and add the cauliflower

3. Add salt, sesame seeds and cook for 4-5 minutes
4. When ready remove from heat, add cilantro and stir to combine
5. Serve with sauce

RICE, KALE AND AVOCADO BOWL

Serves: **2**

Prep Time: **10** Minutes

Cook Time: **20** Minutes

Total Time: **30** Minutes

INGREDIENTS

- 1 cup rice
- 1 garlic clove
- 1 tablespoon rice vinegar
- 2 cups vegetable broth
- pinch of salt
- pinch of pepper
- 2 tablespoons
- 1 bunch kale
- 1 bunch kale
- 1 avocado

DIRECTIONS

1. In a pot stir in broth, rice and garlic
2. Bring to a simmer for and cook until liquid is evaporated
3. When ready toss rice with salt, pepper and vinegar
4. In another books toss kale with olive oil

5. Add kale and avocado slices to the rice
6. Serve when ready

CHICKEN MEATBALLS AND CAULIFLOWER RICE

Serves: **4**
Prep Time: **10**   Minutes

Cook Time: **30**   Minutes

Total Time: **40**   Minutes

INGREDIENTS

- ¼ cup red onion
- 1 lb. ground chicken
- 1 tablespoon mustard
- ¼ tsp black pepper
- 1 tablespoon olive oil
- 1 garlic clove
- ¼ cup parsley
- pinch of salt

SAUCE

- 1 cup parsley
- 1 can coconut milk
- 2 scallions
- zest of 1 lemon
- 1 cup ready-made cauliflower rice

DIRECTIONS

1. In a skillet heat olive oil and sauté onion and garlic for 3-4 minutes
2. Remove sautéed onion and garlic to a bowl
3. Stir in parsley, mustard, chicken, seasoning and mix well
4. Form balls from the mixture and place on a baking sheet
5. Bake at 400 F for 20 minutes
6. When ready remove from the oven and set aside
7. In a blender add all ingredients for the sauce and blend
8. Top the meatballs with sauce and cauliflower rice and serve

PINEAPPLE CHICKEN AND LETTUCE WRAPS

Serves: **2**
Prep Time: **10**   Minutes

Cook Time: **20**   Minutes

Total Time: **30**   Minutes

INGREDIENTS

- 2 cups cooked chicken
- 1 tablespoon olive oil
- ¼ tsp paprika
- 1 tablespoon lime juice
- ¼ tsp garlic powder
- ¼ tsp salt
- 1 cup pineapple cubes
- 8 lettuce wraps

DIRECTIONS

1. In a bowl combine garlic powder, lime juice, paprika, olive oil and lime juice
2. In your lettuce wraps add pineapple cubes, chicken and top with lime mixture
3. Serve when ready

Serves: *4*

Prep Time: *10* Minutes

Cook Time: *35* Minutes

Total Time: *45* Minutes

INGREDIENTS

- 1 lb. potatoes
- 1 tsp lemon juice
- 4 salmon fillets
- ¼ tsp paprika
- 2 tablespoons olive oil

DIRECTIONS

1. Bake the potatoes at 375 F for 20-25 minutes
2. Rub the salmon fillets with paprika and olive oil
3. Bake the fish until golden brown
4. When ready from the oven and serve with baked potatoes and lemon juice

GUT ENERGY BOOSTING BOWL

Serves: *1*
Prep Time: 5   Minutes

Cook Time: 5   Minutes

Total Time: *10* Minutes

INGREDIENTS

- 2 cups kale
- 1 tablespoon olive oil
- 1 avocado
- ¼ cup carrot
- ½ cup beans
- ¼ cup cabbage
- 1 cup baked potatoes

DIRECTIONS

1. In a bowl add all ingredients together
2. Drizzle olive oil and salt and mix well
3. Serve when ready

Serves: *2*
Prep Time: *5*   Minutes

Cook Time: *10* Minutes

Total Time: *15* Minutes

INGREDIENTS

- 2 zucchinis
- pinch of salt
- 2 avocados
- 2 tablespoons olive oil
- 2 eggs
- 1 tablespoon olive oil

DIRECTIONS

1. In a bowl toss the zucchini noodles with olive oil
2. Season and transfer to a baking sheet
3. Crack an egg over each portion
4. Bake for 8-10 minutes at 375 F
5. When ready remove from the oven and serve with avocado slices

CHICKEN WITH BAKED VEGGIES

Serves: **4**
Prep Time: **10** Minutes

Cook Time: **30** Minutes

Total Time: **40** Minutes

INGREDIENTS

- 1 tablespoon olive oil
- 1 tablespoon honey
- 2 red bell peppers
- 2 carrots
- ¼ cup parsley
- 1 lb. chicken breast
- 2 onions

DIRECTIONS

1. Place the chicken onto a baking sheet
2. Add the rest of the ingredients to the chicken breast
3. Drizzle olive oil over chicken and veggies
4. Bake at 375 F for 25-30 minutes or until the vegetables are tender
5. When ready remove from the oven and serve

VEGGIE STIR-FRY

Serves: **2**

Prep Time: **10**   Minutes

Cook Time: **20**   Minutes

Total Time: **30**   Minutes

INGREDIENTS

- 1 tablespoon cornstarch
- 1 garlic clove
- ¼ cup olive oil
- ¼ head broccoli
- ¼ cup show peas
- ½ cup carrots
- ¼ cup green beans
- 1 tablespoon soy sauce
- ½ cup onion

DIRECTIONS

1. In a bowl combine garlic, olive oil, cornstarch and mix well
2. Add the rest of the ingredients and toss to coat
3. In a skillet cook vegetables mixture until tender
4. When ready transfer to a plate garnish with ginger and serve

WALDORF SALAD

Serves: **2**
Prep Time: **5**   Minutes

Cook Time: **5**   Minutes

Total Time: **10**   Minutes

INGREDIENTS

- 1 tablespoon mayonnaise
- 1 tablespoon lemon juice
- 1 apple
- 1 cup red grapes
- ½ cup cranberries
- ½ cup walnuts
- 12 cup celery
- 6 lettuce leaves

DIRECTIONS

1. Combine all ingredients together and mix well
2. Serve with dressing

CRANBERRY SALAD

Serves: **2**

Prep Time: **5**   Minutes

Cook Time: **5**   Minutes

Total Time: *10*   Minutes

INGREDIENTS

- 1 can unsweetened pineapple
- 1 package cherry gelatin
- 1 tablespoon lemon juice
- ½ cup artificial sweetener
- 1 cup cranberries
- 1 orange
- 1 cup celery
- ½ cup pecans

DIRECTIONS

1. Combine all ingredients together and mix well
2. Serve with dressing

ARUGULA SALAD

Serves: *1*
Prep Time: 5   Minutes

Cook Time: 5   Minutes

Total Time: *10*   Minutes

INGREDIENTS

- 2 cups arugula leaves
- ¼ cup cranberries
- ¼ cup honey
- ¼ cup pecans
- 1 cup salad dressing

DIRECTIONS

1. Combine all ingredients together and mix well
2. Serve with dressing

MANDARIN SALAD

Serves: **2**

Prep Time: **10**   Minutes

Cook Time: **20**   Minutes

Total Time: **30**   Minutes

INGREDIENTS

- 2 tsp maple syrup
- 3 tbs oil
- 3 mandarins
- 1 avocado
- 150 g walnuts
- 250 g kale
- 150 g spinach
- 1 lemon
- 150 g Brussels sprouts
- ½ red onion

DIRECTIONS

1. Preheat the oven to 400F
2. Dice the sprouts, red onion, kale and avocado
3. Cut the mandarins
4. Pulse the walnuts just a little using a food processor
5. Mix the walnuts with lemon zest
6. Mix together the maple syrup, oil and lemon juice

7. Add the walnuts to the vegetables, pour the dressing over and
   serve

BEAN FAJITAS

Serves: **2**
Prep Time: **5**   Minutes

Cook Time: **10** Minutes

Total Time: **15** Minutes

INGREDIENTS

- 1 kidney beans can
- Tortillas
- 3 tsp cumin
- 2 tsp garlic powder
- 5 mushrooms
- 2 red peppers
- 2 yellow peppers
- 1 onion

DIRECTIONS

1. Cook the peppers and the onion until caramelized
2. Add the mushrooms, garlic powder and cumin
3. Add the kidney beans after a few minutes when the mushrooms turn brown
4. Cook until soft
5. Heat the tortillas
6. Fill them with the vegetable mixture and serve

TOFU SALAD

Serves: *1*
Prep Time: 5   Minutes

Cook Time: 5   Minutes

Total Time: *10*   Minutes

INGREDIENTS

- 1 pack tofu
- 1 cup chopped vegetables (carrots, cucumber)

DRESSING

- 1 tablespoon sesame oil
- 1 tablespoon mustard
- 1 tablespoon brown rice vinegar
- 1 tablespoon soya sauce

DIRECTIONS

1. Combine all ingredients together and mix well
2. Add salad dressing, toss well and serve

PAD THAI SALAD

Serves: **1**
Prep Time: **5**   Minutes
Cook Time: **5**   Minutes
Total Time: **10** Minutes

INGREDIENTS

- ¼ lb. rice noodles
- 1 red pepper
- 1 onion
- 4 stalks coriander
- ¼ package silken tofu
- 1 oz. roasted peanuts
- Salad dressing

DIRECTIONS

1. Combine all ingredients together and mix well
2. Add salad dressing, toss well and serve

STEW RECIPES

BEEF STEW

Serves: **4**

Prep Time: **15**   Minutes

Cook Time: **45**   Minutes

Total Time: **60**   Minutes

INGREDIENTS

- 2 lb. beef
- 1 tsp salt
- 4 tablespoons olive oil
- 2 red onions
- 2 cloves garlic
- 1 cup white wine
- 2 cups beef broth
- 1 cup water
- 3-4 bay leaves
- ¼ tsp thyme
- 1 lb. potatoes

DIRECTIONS

1. Chop all ingredients in big chunks
2. In a large pot heat olive oil and add ingredients one by one
3. Cook for 5-6 or until slightly brown
4. Add remaining ingredients and cook until tender, 35-45 minutes
5. Season while stirring on low heat
6. When ready remove from heat and serve

IRISH STEW

Serves: **4**

Prep Time: **15** Minutes

Cook Time: **45** Minutes

Total Time: **60** Minutes

INGREDIENTS

- 4-5 slices bacon
- 2 lb. beef
- ¼ cup flour
- ½ tsp black pepper
- 4 carrots
- ½ cup beef broth

DIRECTIONS

1. Chop all ingredients in big chunks
2. In a large pot heat olive oil and add ingredients one by one
3. Cook for 5-6 or until slightly brown
4. Add remaining ingredients and cook until tender, 35-45 minutes
5. Season while stirring on low heat
6. When ready remove from heat and serve

CHICKEN CASSEROLE

Serves: **4**

Prep Time: **10** Minutes

Cook Time: **15** Minutes

Total Time: **25** Minutes

INGREDIENTS

- 1 tablespoon olive oil
- 1 lb. chicken breast
- 1 red onion
- 2 cloves garlic
- 1 tsp paprika
- 4 cups cooked rice
- ¼ cup cranberries
- 1 lb. brussels sprouts
- 1 potato

DIRECTIONS

1. Sauté the veggies and set aside
2. Preheat the oven to 425 F
3. Transfer the sautéed veggies to a baking dish, add remaining ingredients to the baking dish

4. Mix well, add seasoning and place the dish in the oven
5. Bake for 12-15 minutes or until slightly brown
6. When ready remove from the oven and serve

RICE CASSEROLE

Serves: **4**

Prep Time: **10**   Minutes

Cook Time: **15**   Minutes

Total Time: **25**   Minutes

INGREDIENTS

- 2 cups cooked rice
- 1 red onion
- ¼ cup olive oil
- 1 can mushroom soup
- 2 lb. chicken thighs
- 2 tablespoons butter
- 1 clove garlic
- 1 tablespoon parsley

DIRECTIONS

1. Sauté the veggies and set aside
2. Preheat the oven to 425 F
3. Transfer the sautéed veggies to a baking dish, add remaining ingredients to the baking dish
4. Mix well, add seasoning and place the dish in the oven
5. Bake for 12-15 minutes or until slightly brown
6. When ready remove from the oven and serve

PIZZA RECIPES

MUSHROOM PIZZA

Serves: **2**
Prep Time: **10** Minutes

Cook Time: **30** Minutes

Total Time: **40** Minutes

INGREDIENTS

- 2 button mushrooms
- ½ red onion
- 1 lemon juiced
- 1 tablespoon parsley
- ½ cup ground flax seeds
- 2 tablespoons olive oil
- 1 cup almonds whole
- 1 cup cashews whole
- 1 carrot

DIRECTIONS

1. Preheat oven to 375 F and place a baking sheet
2. In food processor place all the ingredients and blend for 8-10 minutes

3. Pour the mixture on the baking sheet and bake for 15-20 minutes until golden
4. Remove from the oven and serve

CASSEROLE PIZZA

Serves: *6-8*

Prep Time: *10*   Minutes

Cook Time: *15*   Minutes

Total Time: *25*   Minutes

INGREDIENTS

- 1 pizza crust
- ½ cup tomato sauce
- ¼ black pepper
- 1 cup zucchini slices
- 1 cup mozzarella cheese
- 1 cup olives

DIRECTIONS

1. Spread tomato sauce on the pizza crust
2. Place all the toppings on the pizza crust
3. Bake the pizza at 425 F for 12-15 minutes
4. When ready remove pizza from the oven and serve

SECOND COOKBOOK

SOUP RECIPES

CAULIFLOWER SOUP

Serves: **4**

Prep Time: **10** Minutes

Cook Time: **20** Minutes

Total Time: **30** Minutes

INGREDIENTS

- 1 tablespoon olive oil
- 1 lb. cauliflower
- ¼ red onion
- ½ cup all-purpose flour
- ¼ tsp salt
- ¼ tsp pepper
- 1 can vegetable broth
- 1 cup heavy cream

DIRECTIONS

1. In a saucepan heat olive oil and sauté cauliflower until tender
2. Add remaining ingredients to the saucepan and bring to a boil
3. When all the vegetables are tender transfer to a blender and blend until smooth
4. Pour soup into bowls, garnish with parsley and serve

Serves: **4**

Prep Time: **10** Minutes

Cook Time: **20** Minutes

Total Time: **30** Minutes

INGREDIENTS

- 1 tablespoon olive oil
- 1 lb. zucchini
- 2 tablespoons garlic
- ¼ red onion
- ½ cup all-purpose flour
- ¼ tsp salt
- ¼ tsp pepper
- 1 can vegetable broth
- 1 cup heavy cream

DIRECTIONS

1. In a saucepan heat olive oil and sauté garlic until tender
2. Add remaining ingredients to the saucepan and bring to a boil
3. When all the vegetables are tender transfer to a blender and blend until smooth
4. Pour soup into bowls, garnish with parsley and serve

LEEK SOUP

Serves: **4**
Prep Time: **10** Minutes

Cook Time: **20** Minutes

Total Time: **30** Minutes

INGREDIENTS

- 1 tablespoon olive oil
- 1 lb. spinach
- ¼ red onion
- ½ cup all-purpose flour
- ¼ tsp salt
- ¼ tsp pepper
- 1 can vegetable broth
- 1 cup heavy cream
- 2 leeks

DIRECTIONS

1. In a saucepan heat olive oil and sauté leek until tender
2. Add remaining ingredients to the saucepan and bring to a boil
3. When all the vegetables are tender transfer to a blender and blend until smooth
4. Pour soup into bowls, garnish with parsley and serve

CARROT SOUP

Serves: **4**

Prep Time: **10**   Minutes

Cook Time: **20**   Minutes

Total Time: **30**   Minutes

INGREDIENTS

- 1 tablespoon olive oil
- 1 lb. carrots
- ¼ red onion
- ½ cup all-purpose flour
- ¼ tsp salt
- ¼ tsp pepper
- 1 can vegetable broth
- 1 cup heavy cream

DIRECTIONS

1. In a saucepan heat olive oil and sauté carrots until tender
2. Add remaining ingredients to the saucepan and bring to a boil
3. When all the vegetables are tender transfer to a blender and blend until smooth
4. Pour soup into bowls, garnish with parsley and serve

CELERY SOUP

Serves: **4**

Prep Time: **10**   Minutes

Cook Time: **20**   Minutes

Total Time: **30**   Minutes

INGREDIENTS

- 1 tablespoon olive oil
- ¼ red onion
- ½ cup all-purpose flour
- ¼ tsp salt
- ¼ tsp pepper
- 1 can vegetable broth
- 1 cup heavy cream
- 1 cup celery

DIRECTIONS

1. In a saucepan heat olive oil and sauté onion until tender
2. Add remaining ingredients to the saucepan and bring to a boil
3. When all the vegetables are tender transfer to a blender and blend until smooth
4. Pour soup into bowls, garnish with parsley and serve

GREEN PESTO PASTA

Serves: **2**

Prep Time: **5**   Minutes

Cook Time: **15**   Minutes

Total Time: **20**   Minutes

INGREDIENTS

- 4 oz. spaghetti
- 2 cups basil leaves
- 2 garlic cloves
- ¼ cup olive oil
- 2 tablespoons parmesan cheese
- ½ tsp black pepper

DIRECTIONS

1. Bring water to a boil and add pasta
2. In a blend add parmesan cheese, basil leaves, garlic and blend
3. Add olive oil, pepper and blend again
4. Pour pesto onto pasta and serve when ready

FIESTA SHRIMP

Serves: **2**
Prep Time: **10** Minutes

Cook Time: **10** Minutes

Total Time: **20** Minutes

INGREDIENTS

- 3 oz. shrimp
- ½ cup zucchini
- ½ cup fiesta garden salsa
- ½ oz. Monterey Jack cheese
- cilantro
- 1 tortilla

DIRECTIONS

1. In a bowl add zucchini, shrimp and salsa
2. Microwave for 4-5 minutes, remove and add grated cheese
3. Sprinkle cilantro and pour mixture over tortilla
4. Serve when ready

DIJON VINAIGRETTE

Serves: **2**

Prep Time: **5**   Minutes

Cook Time: **5**   Minutes

Total Time: **10**   Minutes

INGREDIENTS

- 2 tablespoons red wine vinegar
- 1 tablespoon water
- 1 tablespoon olive oil
- 1 tsp Dijon mustard
- ½ tsp garlic powder

DIRECTIONS

1. **In a bowl mix all ingredients**
2. **Chill overnight and serve**

COTTAGE CHEESE CASSEROLE

Serves: **3**

Prep Time: **10** Minutes

Cook Time: **50** Minutes

Total Time: **60** Minutes

INGREDIENTS

- 2 eggs
- 2 cups cottage cheese
- 1 red onion
- 1 pinch of pepper

DIRECTIONS

1. In a bowl mix all ingredients and pour into a casserole dish
2. Bake at 325 for 50 minutes
3. Remove and serve

FRENCH DRESSING

Serves: **2**

Prep Time: **5** Minutes

Cook Time: **5** Minutes

Total Time: **10** Minutes

INGREDIENTS

- ½ cup ketchup
- ¼ cup oil
- ¼ cup white vinegar
- 1 tsp lemon juice
- dash of pepper

DIRECTIONS

1. In a bowl mix all ingredients
2. Chill overnight and serve

TAPENADE

Serves: **4**

Prep Time: **10**   Minutes

Cook Time: **10**   Minutes

Total Time: **20**   Minutes

INGREDIENTS

- ½ cup Kalamata olives
- 1 tsp capers
- ½ cup olive oil
- 1 tablespoon balsamic vinegar

DIRECTIONS

1. In a bowl chop olive and mix with crushed garlic
2. Add the rest of ingredients and mix well
3. Chill for 1-2 hours serve with asparagus or vegetables

MUSHROOM BACON

Serves: **3**

Prep Time: **10** Minutes

Cook Time: **10** Minutes

Total Time: **20** Minutes

INGREDIENTS

- 1 tablespoon oil
- 1 packet Portobello mushroom
- ½ cup maple syrup
- 1 tablespoon liquid smoke
- pinch of salt
- pinch of pepper

DIRECTIONS

1. In a bowl mix marinate the mushroom slices, mix with liquid smoke, maple syrup salt, and pepper
2. Cut the mushrooms into strips and marinade for 12-15 minutes
3. In a skillet cook mushrooms for 3-5 minutes or until browned
4. Remove, add lettuce, sliced tomato and serve

ZUCCHINI CASSEROLE

Serves: **4**

Prep Time: **10**   Minutes

Cook Time: **1**   Hour 30 Minutes

Total Time: **1**   Hour 30 Minutes

INGREDIENTS

- 2 lb. zucchini
- 1 onion
- ½ cup rice
- 1 can mushroom soup
- 2 beaten eggs
- 2 tablespoons butter
- 1 cup cheddar cheese

DIRECTIONS

1. Preheat the oven 325 F
2. In a bowl mix all ingredients
3. Pour mixture into a casserole dish
4. Top with grated cheese

NOODLES WITH PARMESAN CHEESE

Serves: **4**

Prep Time: **10** Minutes

Cook Time: **30** Minutes

Total Time: **40** Minutes

INGREDIENTS

- 1 lb. noodles
- 1 cup parmesan cheese
- 2 cloves garlic
- 3 tablespoons coriander
- 5 tablespoons olive oil
- ¾ tsp salt
- ¼ tsp pepper

DIRECTIONS

1. Cook noodles according to directions and place in a bowl
2. Chop coriander and place in a bowl with crushed garlic
3. Mix with remaining ingredients, stir into the noodles
4. Serve when ready

BALSAMIC CHICKEN

Serves: **4**

Prep Time: **10**   Minutes

Cook Time: **2**   Hours 30 Minutes

Total Time: **2**   Hours 40 Hours

INGREDIENTS

- 3 chicken breasts
- ¼ cup olive oil
- ¼ cup balsamic vinegar
- 1 clove garlic

DIRECTIONS

1. In a bowl, add all ingredients
2. Add chicken and marinade for 3-4 hours
3. Grill and serve with vegetables

STEAMED SALMON

Serves: **4**

Prep Time: **10**   Minutes

Cook Time: **30**   Minutes

Total Time: **40**   Minutes

INGREDIENTS

- 3 salmon fillets
- ½ tsp dill weed
- ½ tsp parsley
- salt

DIRECTIONS

1. Season the salmon with pepper and parsley
2. Place each fillet on the grill at 325 F for 30 minutes
3. Remove and serve with vegetables

ROASTED POTATOES

Serves: **4**

Prep Time: **10**   Minutes

Cook Time: **20**   Minutes

Total Time: **30**   Minutes

INGREDIENTS

- 1 red potato wedges
- 1 tablespoon rosemary
- 2 garlic cloves
- 1 tablespoon olive oil
- ¼ tsp onion powder
- ½ tsp salt
- ½ tsp pepper

DIRECTIONS

1. In a bowl mix potato wedges and the rest of the ingredients
2. Toss to coat the potato wedges and place on a baking sheet
3. Bake for 20-25 minutes or until tender
4. Remove and serve

Serves: *1*
Prep Time: *5*   Minutes

Cook Time: *5*   Minutes

Total Time: *10* Minutes

INGREDIENTS

- 1 lb beef
- 1 package taco seasoning
- 1 iceberg lettuce
- 3 tomatoes
- 1 cup cheese
- 1/3 cup corn
- 1 bunch scallions

DIRECTIONS

1. Brown the beef, then season
2. In a bowl mix all ingredients and mix well
3. Serve with dressing

CHICKEN SALAD

Serves: **6**

Prep Time: **5**   Minutes

Cook Time: **5**   Minutes

Total Time: **10**   Minutes

INGREDIENTS

- 3 cups chicken
- 1 cup pecans
- ½ cup Greek yogurt
- 3 celery stalks
- 1/3 cup mayonnaise
- 3 tsp mustard
- 2 tsp vinegar
- 1 tsp salt
- Black pepper
- 1/3 cup red onion
- ¼ cup parsley

DIRECTIONS

1. Toast the pecans
2. Cook the chicken
3. Allow the pecans to cool, then chop

4. In a bowl mix all ingredients and mix well
5. Serve with dressing

CRANBERRY PECAN SALAD

Serves: **2**

Prep Time: 5   Minutes

Cook Time: 5   Minutes

Total Time: **10**   Minutes

INGREDIENTS

- 1 cup cooked chicken breast
- 1 tablespoon pecans
- 2 tablespoons cranberries
- ¼ cup red onion
- 2 tablespoons Greek yogurt
- 1 tsp dried thyme
- 1 cup salad dressing

DIRECTIONS

1. In a bowl combine all ingredients together and mix well
2. Serve with dressing

Serves: 2

Prep Time: 5   Minutes

Cook Time: 5   Minutes

Total Time: *10*   Minutes

INGREDIENTS

- 4 cups romaine lettuce
- 2 pears
- ½ cup cranberries
- ¼ cup pecans
- ¼ cup red onion
- 4 slices turkey bacon
- ¼ cup cheese

DIRECTIONS

1. In a bowl combine all ingredients together and mix well
2. Serve with dressing

WATERMELON SALAD

Serves: 2

Prep Time: 5   Minutes

Cook Time: 5   Minutes

Total Time: *10*   Minutes

INGREDIENTS

- 5 cups watermelon
- ½ cup feta cheese
- ¼ red onion
- ¼ black olives
- 3 tablespoons rice vinegar

DIRECTIONS

1. In a bowl combine all ingredients together and mix well
2. Serve with dressing

Serves: 2

Prep Time: 5   Minutes

Cook Time: 5   Minutes

Total Time: 10   Minutes

INGREDIENTS

- 4 cups white potato
- 1 pinch salt
- 2 tablespoons olive oil
- ¼ cup corn
- ½ cup black beans
- 2 tablespoons lemon juice

DIRECTIONS

1. In a bowl combine all ingredients together and mix well
2. Serve with dressing

SOUTHWESTERN SALAD

Serves: **2**

Prep Time: **5**   Minutes

Cook Time: **5**   Minutes

Total Time: **10** Minutes

INGREDIENTS

- 4 cups cooked white potato
- 2 tablespoons olive oil
- ¼ cup red bell pepper
- ¼ cup red onion
- ½ cup corn
- ¼ cup cilantro
- 1 tsp garlic
- 1 cup salad dressing

DIRECTIONS

1. In a bowl combine all ingredients together and mix well
2. Serve with dressing

TOMATO SALAD

Serves: 2

Prep Time: 5   Minutes

Cook Time: 5   Minutes

Total Time: *10*   Minutes

INGREDIENTS

- 2 cups watermelon
- ¼ red onion
- ¼ cup fete cheese
- 2 cups tomatoes
- 1 tablespoon basil
- 1 cup salad dressing

DIRECTIONS

1. In a bowl combine all ingredients together and mix well
2. Serve with dressing

MELON SALAD

Serves: **2**

Prep Time: **5**   Minutes

Cook Time: **5**   Minutes

Total Time: **10** Minutes

INGREDIENTS

- 1 package baby spinach
- 1 cup cantaloupe
- 1 cucumber
- 1 cup red onion
- 2 tablespoons honey

DIRECTIONS

1. In a bowl combine all ingredients together and mix well
2. Serve with dressing

Serves: *2*
Prep Time: *10*   Minutes

Cook Time: *20*   Minutes

Total Time: *30*   Minutes

INGREDIENTS

- ½ lb. red cabbage
- 1 tablespoon olive oil
- ½ red onion
- 2 eggs
- ¼ tsp salt
- 2 oz. cheddar cheese
- 1 garlic clove
- ¼ tsp dill

DIRECTIONS

1. In a bowl whisk eggs with salt and cheese
2. In a frying pan heat olive oil and pour egg mixture
3. Add remaining ingredients and mix well
4. Serve when ready

KALE FRITATTA

Serves: **2**

Prep Time: **10**   Minutes

Cook Time: **20**   Minutes

Total Time: **30**   Minutes

INGREDIENTS

- 1 cup kale
- 1 tablespoon olive oil
- ½ red onion
- ¼ tsp salt
- 2 eggs
- 2 oz. cheddar cheese
- 1 garlic clove
- ¼ tsp dill

DIRECTIONS

1. In a skillet sauté kale until tender
2. In a bowl whisk eggs with salt and cheese
3. In a frying pan heat olive oil and pour egg mixture
4. Add remaining ingredients and mix well
5. When ready serve with sautéed kale

BRUSSEL SPROUTS FRITATTA

Serves: 2
Prep Time: **10** Minutes

Cook Time: **20** Minutes

Total Time: **30** Minutes

INGREDIENTS

- 1 cup brussel sprouts
- 1 tablespoon olive oil
- ½ red onion
- ¼ tsp salt
- 2 eggs
- 2 oz. parmesan cheese
- 1 garlic clove
- ¼ tsp dill

DIRECTIONS

1. In a bowl whisk eggs with salt and cheese
2. In a frying pan heat olive oil and pour egg mixture
3. Add remaining ingredients and mix well
4. Serve when ready

BROCCOLI FRITATTA

Serves: **2**

Prep Time: **10** Minutes

Cook Time: **20** Minutes

Total Time: **30** Minutes

INGREDIENTS

- 1 cup broccoli
- 1 tablespoon olive oil
- ½ red onion
- ¼ tsp salt
- 2 eggs
- 2 oz. cheddar cheese
- 1 garlic clove
- ¼ tsp dill

DIRECTIONS

1. In a skillet sauté broccoli until tender
2. In a bowl whisk eggs with salt and cheese
3. In a frying pan heat olive oil and pour egg mixture
4. Add remaining ingredients and mix well
5. When ready serve with sautéed broccoli

SPAGHETI SQUASH

Serves: **2**
Prep Time: **5**   Minutes

Cook Time: **15**   Minutes

Total Time: **20**   Minutes

INGREDIENTS

- 1 spaghetti squash

DIRECTIONS

1. Cut the spaghetti squash in half and remove seeds
2. Spiralize the squash and set aside
3. Fill a container with water and place the squash side down in a container
4. Microwave for 5-6 minutes
5. Serve when ready

SPICY MUSSELS

Serves: **4**

Prep Time: **10** Minutes

Cook Time: **20** Minutes

Total Time: **30** Minutes

INGREDIENTS

- 2 shallots
- 2 garlic cloves
- 2 tablespoons chilies
- 1 cup water
- 2 tablespoon soy sauce
- 2 lb. mussels

DIRECTIONS

1. Place all ingredients in a pot and bring to a boil
2. Simmer on medium heat for 12-15 minutes
3. Cover with a lid and cook until mussels cover up
4. Serve when ready

SHRIMP FAJITAS

Serves: *4*

Prep Time: *10*   Minutes

Cook Time: *20*   Minutes

Total Time: *30*   Minutes

INGREDIENTS

- 2 tsp Chile powder
- 2 tsp salt
- 1 tsp cumin
- 1 tsp onion powder
- 2 tablespoons lime juice
- 2 lb. shrimp
- 1 green pepper
- 1 red onion

DIRECTIONS

1. Mix all spices together and place fajita aside
2. Toss the shrimp with fajita seasoning and let marinate for a couple of minutes
3. In a skillet heat oil and cook shrimp until soft
4. When ready remove from the skillet and serve

GARLIC CLAMS

Serves: *2*

Prep Time: *10*   Minutes

Cook Time: *20*   Minutes

Total Time: *30*   Minutes

INGREDIENTS

- 1 cup water
- 2 tablespoons lemon juice
- 2 garlic cloves
- 1 tsp thyme
- 1 lb. clams
- ¼ tsp salt

DIRECTIONS

1. In a skillet heat olive oil and sauté garlic, onion and thyme for 4-5 minutes
2. Add water, salt, lemon juice and clams
3. Cover with a lid and cook until shells open up
4. Serve when ready

CROCKPOT CHICKEN

Serves: *6-8*

Prep Time: *10*   Minutes

Cook Time: 5   Hours

Total Time: 5   Hours 10 Minutes

INGREDIENTS

- 1 chicken
- 1 tsp paprika
- 1 tsp salt
- 1 tsp pepper
- 1 tsp garlic powder
- 1 tsp basil
- 1 tsp oregano
- 4-5 lemon slices
- 4-5 potato slices

DIRECTIONS

1. Mix all spices together and rub the chicken with the mixture
2. Stuff the chicken with lemon and potato slices
3. Place the chicken into the slow cooker and cook on medium for 4-5 hours
4. When ready remove from the slow cooker and serve

ROASTED SQUASH

Serves: **3-4**
Prep Time: **10**   Minutes

Cook Time: **20**   Minutes

Total Time: **30**   Minutes

INGREDIENTS

- 2 delicata squashes
- 2 tablespoons olive oil
- 1 tsp curry powder
- 1 tsp salt

DIRECTIONS

1. Preheat the oven to 400 F
2. Cut everything in half lengthwise
3. Toss everything with olive oil and place onto a prepared baking sheet
4. Roast for 18-20 minutes at 400 F or until golden brown
5. When ready remove from the oven and serve

CUCUMBER CHIPS

Serves: **2**

Prep Time: **10** Minutes

Cook Time: **20** Minutes

Total Time: **30** Minutes

INGREDIENTS

- 1 lb. cucumber
- 1 tsp salt
- 1 tsp smoked paprika
- 1 tablespoon olive oil

DIRECTIONS

1. Preheat the oven to 425 F
2. In a bowl toss everything with olive oil and seasoning
3. Spread everything onto a prepared baking sheet
4. Bake for 8-10 minutes or until crisp
5. When ready remove from the oven and serve

SQUASH CHIPS

Serves: **2**
Prep Time: **10**   Minutes

Cook Time: **20**   Minutes

Total Time: **30**   Minutes

INGREDIENTS

- 1 lb. squash
- 1 tsp salt
- 1 tsp smoked paprika
- 1 tablespoon olive oil

DIRECTIONS

1. Preheat the oven to 425 F
2. In a bowl toss everything with olive oil and seasoning
3. Spread everything onto a prepared baking sheet
4. Bake for 8-10 minutes or until crisp
5. When ready remove from the oven and serve

PIZZA

ZUCCHINI PIZZA

Serves: **6-8**
Prep Time: **10**   Minutes

Cook Time: **15**   Minutes

Total Time: **25**   Minutes

INGREDIENTS

- 1 pizza crust
- ½ cup tomato sauce
- ¼ black pepper
- 1 cup zucchini slices
- 1 cup mozzarella cheese
- 1 cup olives

DIRECTIONS

1. Spread tomato sauce on the pizza crust
2. Place all the toppings on the pizza crust
3. Bake the pizza at 425 F for 12-15 minutes
4. When ready remove pizza from the oven and serve

CHICKEN PIZZA

Serves: *2*
Prep Time: *10* Minutes

Cook Time: *20* Minutes

Total Time: *30* Minutes

INGREDIENTS

- 1 ready-made pizza crust
- 1 tsp olive oil
- 1 cup onion
- 14 cup red pepper strips
- 1 cup chicken
- ¼ cup barbecue sauce
- 1 cup mozzarella cheese
- topping of any choice

DIRECTIONS

1. Preheat the oven to 425 F
2. In a frying pan add pepper strips, onion, chicken and cook on low heat
3. Cook until ready and remove from heat
4. Place crust on a cookie sheet and spread barbecue sauce, and the rest of ingredients on the crust
5. Top with mozzarella and bake for 12-15 minutes

CIABATTA PIZZA

Serves: *2*
Prep Time: *10*   Minutes

Cook Time: *20*   Minutes

Total Time: *30*   Minutes

INGREDIENTS

- 1 loaf ciabatta
- 1 cup tomato sauce
- 1 zucchini
- ½ cup mushrooms
- 1 cup mozzarella cheese
- 1 tablespoon basil

DIRECTIONS

1. Preheat the oven to 375 F
2. Cum ciabatta lengthwise and place on a cookie sheet
3. Spread sauce, zucchini, mushrooms on each one and top with mozzarella
4. Sprinkle basil, bake for 12-15 minutes, remove and serve

SHRIMP PIZZA

Serves: **2**

Prep Time: **10** Minutes

Cook Time: **20** Minutes

Total Time: **30** Minutes

INGREDIENTS

- 13 oz. pizza dough
- 1 tablespoon cornmeal
- ¼ cup ricotta cheese
- 1 lb. shrimp
- 5 cloves garlic
- 1 cup mozzarella cheese
- 1 tablespoon dried basil

DIRECTIONS

1. Preheat the oven to 375 F
2. In a baking pan sprinkle cornmeal and add the pizza dough, bake for 6-8 minutes
3. Remove and cover pizza with mozzarella, ricotta, garlic and sprinkle with basil
4. Bake for 12-15 minutes, remove and serve

THIRD COOKBOOK

FRENCH TOAST

Serves: 2

Prep Time: 5   minutes

Cook Time: 5   minutes

Total Time: *10*   minutes

INGREDIENTS

- 1 ½ tsp cinnamon
- 4 slices bread
- 2 tsp vanilla
- 4 eggs
- 3 tbs milk

DIRECTIONS

1. Whisk together the eggs, milk, vanilla and cinnamon in a bowl
2. Soak the bread into the mixture
3. Heat a greased pan
4. Cook the soaked bread for about 2 minutes per side until golden
5. Serve immediately

Serves: *4*

Prep Time: *10*   Minutes

Cook Time: *15*   Minutes

Total Time: *25*   Minutes

INGREDIENTS

- 1 cup quinoa
- 2 tbs almonds
- 3 tbs coconut
- 1/3 tsp cinnamon
- 1 cup strawberries
- 2 cups milk
- 3 tbs maple syrup

DIRECTIONS

1. Place the quinoa and the milk in a pot and bring to a boil
2. Reduce the heat and simmer for at least 10 minutes
3. Stir in 2 extra tbs of milk, maple syrup and cinnamon
4. Divide into bowls and top with strawberries, coconut and almonds

CHEESE SANDWICH

Serves: **1**

Prep Time: **5**   Minutes

Cook Time: **5**   Minutes

Total Time: **10** Minutes

INGREDIENTS

- 4 slices tomato
- 1 oz cheese
- 2 tbs mayonnaise
- 1 slice bread
- 1 can sardines
- ¼ tsp turmeric
- A pinch salt
- A pinch black pepper

DIRECTIONS

1. Mix the sardines, mayonnaise, turmeric and salt
2. Toast the bread
3. Spread the mixture over the bread
4. Top with tomato slices and then with the cheese slices
5. Broil in the preheated oven for 2 minutes
6. Serve topped with black pepper

Serves: **2**
Prep Time: **5**   Minutes

Cook Time: **5**   Minutes

Total Time: **10**   Minutes

INGREDIENTS

- 2 cups coconut milk
- Raspberries
- 1 banana
- ½ cup rolled oats
- Handful spinach leaves
- 1/3 cup chia seeds
- ½ mango
- 1 pear

DIRECTIONS

1. Place the banana, spinach and coconut milk in a food processor and pulse until smooth
2. Stir in the chia seeds and the oats, mixing well
3. Refrigerate covered overnight
4. Peel and dice the mango
5. Top the oats with mango, pear and raspberries
6. Serve when ready

Serves: **2**

Prep Time: **5**   Minutes

Cook Time: **5**   Minutes

Total Time: **10** Minutes

INGREDIENTS

- 1/3 cup black beans
- 3 tbs salsa
- 1 scallion
- 2 tbs cilantro
- 2 eggs
- 1 tortilla
- ½ avocado
- 1 tomato
- 1/3 cup shredded cheese

DIRECTIONS

1. Cook the salsa, black beans, cilantro and scallions for about 2 minutes
2. Add in the eggs and cook until set
3. Heat the tortilla
4. Spoon the cooked mixture onto the tortilla, then top with diced avocado, tomato and cheese

5. Roll-up the tortilla and cut in half
6. Serve immediately

BANANA BREAD

Serves: **12**

Prep Time: **10** Minutes

Cook Time: **50** Minutes

Total Time: **60** Minutes

INGREDIENTS

- 2 bananas
- 2 eggs
- 3 tsp vanilla
- 1 cup flour
- 1 tsp cinnamon
- ½ tsp nutmeg
- 1 cup grape juice
- 1 tsp baking soda
- 1/3 cup walnuts
- ¼ cup oil
- 2 tbs baking powder
- 1/3 cup oat bran
- 1/3 cup oats

DIRECTIONS

1. Mix the banana, oil, eggs, vanilla and eggs in a blender and pulse until smooth

2. Mix the flaxseed, oats, flour, nutmeg, cinnamon, baking soda and baking powder in a separate bowl and stir well

3. Stir in the banana mixture into the flour mixture, mixing gently

4. Fold in the walnuts

5. Spoon the batter into a greased pan

6. Cook in the preheated oven for 50 minutes at 350F

7. Allow to cool, then serve

BLUEBERRY PANCAKES

Serves: **4**

Prep Time: **10** Minutes

Cook Time: **10** Minutes

Total Time: **20** Minutes

INGREDIENTS

- 2 cup blueberries
- 2 tsp baking powder
- 1 ½ cup flour
- 2 tsp baking soda
- 2 eggs
- 1/3 cup oil
- 1/3 cup grape juice
- 1/3 tsp vanilla
- 1/3 cup oats
- 1 ½ cups buttermilk

DIRECTIONS

1. Mix together the flour, baking powder and baking soda and the oats
2. Whisk the eggs with ¼ cup oil, grape juice and vanilla in a separate bowl
3. Pour the buttermilk and the egg mixture over the dry ingredients

4. Stir to combine, then fold in the blueberries
5. Cook the pancakes in 1 tbs of hot oil
6. Cook on both sides until golden brown
7. Serve topped with maple syrup

NUTS AND DATES BARS

Serves: *8*
Prep Time: *10*   Minutes

Cook Time: *20*   Minutes

Total Time: *30*   Minutes

INGREDIENTS

- 4 oz butter
- 1 oz sesame seeds
- 1 oz flaxseeds
- 2 oz nuts
- 3 oz rolled oats
- 1 egg
- 3 oz
- 4 oz dates
- 3 tbs syrup

DIRECTIONS

1. Mix the butter and the syrup together
2. Beat the eggs and mix with the almonds
3. Stir in the egg mixture into the butter mixture
4. Mix in the remaining ingredients
5. Pour into a greased baking tin and bake for at least 20 minutes

APPLE PORRIDGE

Serves: 2
Prep Time: 5   Minutes

Cook Time: 10   Minutes

Total Time: 15   Minutes

INGREDIENTS

- Grated apple
- 1 tsp flaxseed
- Handful sultanas
- 1 ½ tsp maca
- Apple puree
- Nuts
- Honey
- Handful cranberries
- 1 banana
- 1 dollop yogurt
- Blueberries
- Raspberries

DIRECTIONS

1. Prepare the porridge as you desire
2. Stir in the remaining ingredients
3. Cook over gentle heat until thick

Serves: *2*

Prep Time: *10*   Minutes

Cook Time: *20*   Minutes

Total Time: *30*   Minutes

INGREDIENTS

- 1/3 cup sunflower, pumpkin, sesame and chia seeds
- 1 cup pecan nuts
- 2 cups rolled oats
- 1/3 cup cranberries
- 1/3 cup almonds
- 1/3 cup coconut oil
- 1/3 cup peanut butter
- 1/3 cup water
- ½ cup honey

DIRECTIONS

1. Mix the dry ingredients together
2. Mix the coconut oil, honey, water and peanut butter together in a bowl
3. Mix in the wet ingredients into the dry ingredients until combined
4. Pour the mixture into a lined baking sheet

5. Bake in the preheated oven at 350F for at least 15 minutes
6. Allow to cool, then serve

BLUEBERRY FRENCH TOAST

Serves: **6**

Prep Time: **10**   Minutes

Cook Time: **50**   Minutes

Total Time: **60**   Minutes

INGREDIENTS

- 1 cup blueberries
- 4 eggs
- 1 cup coconut milk
- ¼ cup honey
- 1 tsp ground cinnamon
- 1 tablespoon vanilla extract
- 1 zucchini slice "bread"

DIRECTIONS

1. In a baking dish add zucchini "bread" cubes and blueberries
2. In a bowl mix honey, coconut milk, eggs, cinnamon and vanilla extract
3. Pour egg mixture over bread and bake at 325 F for 45 minutes

PUMPKIN MUFFINS

Serves: *8*

Prep Time: *10*   Minutes

Cook Time: *30*   Minutes

Total Time: *40*   Minutes

INGREDIENTS

- 5 eggs
- ½ cup pumpkin puree
- ½ tsp baking soda
- ½ cup almond flour
- ¼ tsp salt

TOPPING

- 1 tablespoon unsweetened coconut flakes
- 1 tablespoon cinnamon

DIRECTIONS

1. In a blender add pumpkin, combine eggs and blend until smooth
2. Add baking soda, coconut flour, baking soda, and blend until smooth
3. Divide batter between 8-10 muffin cups
4. In a blender add topping ingredients and blend until smooth
5. Bake muffins for 25 minutes at 325 F, remove and pour topping over

Serves: *2*
Prep Time: *10* Minutes

Cook Time: *20* Minutes

Total Time: *30* Minutes

INGREDIENTS

- 1 cup SCD Safe homemade yogurt
- 1-quart almond milk

DIRECTIONS

1. In a pot heat milk
2. Place yogurt in mason jar
3. Place ½ cup of milk into jar and stir until smooth
4. Pour remaining milk into mason jar
5. Refrigerate overnight and serve in the morning

CRANBERRY WALNUT SCONES

Serves: *8*

Prep Time: *10*   Minutes

Cook Time: *20*   Minutes

Total Time: *30*   Minutes

INGREDIENTS

- 2 cups almond flour
- ½ tsp baking soda
- 1 tablespoon orange zest
- ½ cup walnuts chopped
- 1 egg
- 2 tablespoons unsweetened coconut flakes

DIRECTIONS

1. In a blender add all ingredients and blend until smooth
2. Transfer dough into a to the oven and bake at 325 F for 15-16 minutes

PIZZA MUFFINS

Serves: *8*
Prep Time: *10* Minutes

Cook Time: *30* Minutes

Total Time: *40* Minutes

INGREDIENTS

- 1 cup almond flour
- ½ tsp salt
- ½ cup cheddar cheese
- ½ cup parmesan cheese
- ½ tsp baking soda
- 4 eggs
- ½ cup tomato sauce

DIRECTIONS

1. In a blender add all ingredients and blend until smooth
2. Line a 12 muffin cups with paper and pour batter into each cup
3. Bake at 325 for 25 minutes
4. Remove from oven and add sauce on each muffin

CINNAMON CAKE

Serves: **4**

Prep Time: **10** Minutes

Cook Time: **30** Minutes

Total Time: **40** Minutes

INGREDIENTS

- 2 cups almond flour
- ½ cup honey
- 2 eggs
- ¼ tsp salt
- ½ tsp baking soda
- ¼ cup coconut oil

TOPPING

- ¼ cup coconut oil
- 2 tablespoons cinnamon
- ½ cup almonds

DIRECTIONS

1. In a blender add all ingredients and blend until smooth
2. Spread the batter into baking dish
3. In a bowl add the topping ingredients and mix well
4. Pour topping over cake batter

5. Bake the cake for 30 minutes at 325

Serves: **4**

Prep Time: **10** Minutes

Cook Time: **30** Minutes

Total Time: **40** Minutes

INGREDIENTS

- 2 cups almond flour
- ½ cup honey
- 1 egg
- ¼ tsp salt
- 1 tablespoon orange zest
- ¼ tsp baking soda

DIRECTIONS

1. In a blender add all the ingredients and blend until smooth
2. Chill dough in freezer for 15 minutes
3. Transfer to a parchment paper line baking sheet
4. Bake at 325 F for 30 minutes

CREPES

Serves: **4**

Prep Time: **10** Minutes

Cook Time: **30** Minutes

Total Time: **40** Minutes

INGREDIENTS

- 2 tablespoons coconut flour
- 3 eggs
- 1 tablespoon coconut oil
- ½ cup water
- 2 tablespoons coconut oil for cooking

DIRECTIONS

1. In a blender add all ingredients and blend until smooth
2. In a frying pan add coconut oil over medium heat
3. Pour batter onto the skillet and cook 1-2 minutes per side

Serves: **12**

Prep Time: **10** Minutes

Cook Time: **30** Minutes

Total Time: **40** Minutes

INGREDIENTS

- 1 cup almond flour
- 2 tablespoons apple cider (SCD Safe)
- ½ tsp salt
- 5 eggs
- 1 tablespoon coconut flour
- 1 tsp baking soda
- 1 tablespoon onion flakes

DIRECTIONS

1. In a blender add all ingredients and blend until smooth
2. Sprinkle bagels dough with onion flakes
3. Bake at 325 F for 15 minutes, remove and serve

PUMPKING CRANBERRY GRANOLA

Serves: **8**

Prep Time: **10** Minutes

Cook Time: **30** Minutes

Total Time: **40** Minutes

INGREDIENTS

- 1 cup almonds
- 1 cup macadamia nuts
- 1 tablespoon cinnamon
- ½ tsp salt
- ½ cu dried cranberries
- 1 cup pumpkin seeds
- 1 cup roasted pumpkin
- 2 tablespoons honey

DIRECTIONS

1. In a bowl place seeds and nuts, cover with water and soak overnight
2. Drain and rinse the seeds and nuts
3. In a blender add the nuts and seeds and blend until smooth
4. Add in the blender honey, cinnamon, pumpkin puree, salt and blend again
5. Spread mixture into 2 baking sheets

6. Bake at 150 F for 10 hours or until crispy

ORANGE BISCUITS

Serves: **6**

Prep Time: **10**   Minutes

Cook Time: **30**   Minutes

Total Time: **40**   Minutes

INGREDIENTS

- ¼ cup coconut flour
- ¼ tsp salt
- ¼ tsp baking soda
- 4 eggs
- 1 tablespoon orange zest
- ½ cup cranberries

DIRECTIONS

1. In a blender add all the ingredients except cranberries
2. Remove mixture from blender and add cranberries
3. Bake the mixture for 20 minutes at 325 F
4. Remove and cool for 15 minutes before serving

Serves: *6*

Prep Time: *10* Minutes

Cook Time: *30* Minutes

Total Time: *40* Minutes

INGREDIENTS

- 1 cup almond flour
- 1 tablespoon coconut flour
- 1 tsp baking soda
- 1 tablespoon apple cider (SCD safe)
- ½ tsp salt
- 5 eggs

DIRECTIONS

1. In a blender add, salt, almond flour, coconut flour, eggs and vinegar, blend until smooth
2. Place batter in a plastic bag
3. Bake at 325 F for 25 minutes
4. Remove and let it cook before serving

LEMON MUFFINS

Serves: *12*

Prep Time: *10*   Minutes

Cook Time: *20*   Minutes

Total Time: *30*   Minutes

INGREDIENTS

- ½ cup coconut flour
- ½ cup honey
- 1 tablespoon lemon zest
- ½ tsp salt
- ½ tsp baking soda
- 3 eggs

DIRECTIONS

1. In a blender add all the ingredients and blend until smooth
2. Spoon batter into muffin pans
3. Bake for 325 F and 10-15 minutes, remove and serve

Serves: *16*

Prep Time: *10*   Minutes

Cook Time: *30*   Minutes

Total Time: *40*   Minutes

INGREDIENTS

- 1 cup almond flour
- ½ tsp salt
- ½ cup coconut oil
- 1 tablespoon honey
- 1 tablespoon water
- 1 tsp vanilla extract
- ½ cup shredded coconut
- ½ cup pumpkin seeds
- ½ cup almonds
- ½ cup raisins

DIRECTIONS

1. In a blender add all ingredients and blend until smooth
2. Pour dough into a baking dish
3. Bake at 325 F for 20 minutes
4. Remove and serve

MORNING SCONES

Serves: **6**
Prep Time: **10** Minutes

Cook Time: **30** Minutes

Total Time: **40** Minutes

INGREDIENTS

- ½ cup coconut flour
- ½ cup honey
- 5 eggs
- ½ tsp salt
- ½ tsp baking soda
- ¼ tsp vanilla extract

DIRECTIONS

1. In a blender add all ingredients and blend until smooth
2. Scoop batter onto a parchment paper
3. Bake at 325F for 15 minutes
4. Remove, let it cool and serve

PUMPKIN MUFFINS

Serves: *8*

Prep Time: *10* Minutes

Cook Time: *20* Minutes

Total Time: *30* Minutes

INGREDIENTS

- ¼ cup coconut flour
- ½ cup roasted pumpkin
- 1 tablespoon cinnamon
- 1 tablespoon ginger
- 4 eggs
- ½ cup honey
- ¼ tsp salt
- ½ tsp baking soda

DIRECTIONS

1. In a blender add all the ingredients and blend until smooth
2. Transfer batter into a paper lined muffin pan
3. Bake at 325 F for 20 minutes
4. Remove, let it cool and serve

PALEO PORRIDGE

Serves: 2

Prep Time: 10   Minutes

Cook Time: 30   Minutes

Total Time: 40   Minutes

INGREDIENTS

- 2 tablespoons shredded coconut
- 1 tsp cinnamon
- 1 tablespoon chia seeds
- ½ cup walnuts
- ½ tsp salt
- 1 cup boiling water
- 1 tablespoon pumpkin seeds

DIRECTIONS

1. In a blender add all ingredients and blend until smooth
2. Transfer porridge to a bowl
3. Garnish with raisins, shredded coconut and sunflower seeds
4. Serve when ready

TART RECIPES

STRAWBERRY TART

Serves: *6-8*

Prep Time: 25   Minutes

Cook Time: 25   Minutes

Total Time: *50*   Minutes

INGREDIENTS

- pastry sheets
- ½ lb. mascarpone
- 200 ml double cream
- 2 tablespoons sugar
- 2 tablespoons honey
- 2 tablespoons lemon juice
- 1 lb. strawberries

DIRECTIONS

1. Preheat oven to 400 F, unfold pastry sheets and place them on a baking sheet
2. Toss together all ingredients and mix well
3. Spread mixture in a single layer on the pastry sheets
4. Before baking, decorate with your desired fruits
5. Bake at 400 F for 22-25 minutes or until golden brown

HAZELNUT TART

Serves: **6-8**
Prep Time: **25**   Minutes

Cook Time: **25**   Minutes

Total Time: **50**   Minutes

INGREDIENTS

- pastry sheets
- 3 oz. brown sugar
- ¼ lb. hazelnuts
- 100 ml double cream
- 2 tablespoons syrup
- ¼ lb. dark chocolate
- 2 oz. butter

DIRECTIONS

1. Preheat oven to 400 F, unfold pastry sheets and place them on a baking sheet
2. Toss together all ingredients together and mix well
3. Spread mixture in a single layer on the pastry sheets
4. Before baking decorate with your desired fruits
5. Bake at 400 F for 22-25 minutes or until golden brown
6. When ready remove from the oven and serve

PEACH PECAN PIE

Serves: **8-12**

Prep Time: **15**   Minutes

Cook Time: **35**   Minutes

Total Time: **50**   Minutes

INGREDIENTS

- 4-5 cups peaches
- 1 tablespoon preserves
- 1 cup sugar
- 4 small egg yolks
- ¼ cup flour
- 1 tsp vanilla extract

DIRECTIONS

1. Line a pie plate or pie form with pastry and cover the edges of the plate depending on your preference
2. In a bowl combine all pie ingredients together and mix well
3. Pour the mixture over the pastry
4. Bake at 400-425 F for 25-30 minutes or until golden brown
5. When ready remove from the oven and let it rest for 15 minutes

OREO PIE

Serves: *8-12*

Prep Time: *15*   Minutes

Cook Time: *35*   Minutes

Total Time: *50*   Minutes

INGREDIENTS

- pastry sheets
- 6-8 oz. chocolate crumb piecrust
- 1 cup half-and-half
- 1 package instant pudding mix
- 10-12 Oreo cookies
- 10 oz. whipped topping

DIRECTIONS

1. Line a pie plate or pie form with pastry and cover the edges of the plate depending on your preference
2. In a bowl combine all pie ingredients together and mix well
3. Pour the mixture over the pastry
4. Bake at 400-425 F for 25-30 minutes or until golden brown
5. When ready remove from the oven and let it rest for 15 minutes

GRAPEFRUIT PIE

Serves: *8-12*

Prep Time: *15*   Minutes

Cook Time: *35*   Minutes

Total Time: *50*   Minutes

INGREDIENTS

- pastry sheets
- 2 cups grapefruit
- 1 cup brown sugar
- ¼ cup flour
- 5-6 egg yolks
- 5 oz. butter

DIRECTIONS

1. Line a pie plate or pie form with pastry and cover the edges of the plate depending on your preference
2. In a bowl combine all pie ingredients together and mix well
3. Pour the mixture over the pastry
4. Bake at 400-425 F for 25-30 minutes or until golden brown
5. When ready remove from the oven and let it rest for 15 minutes

TURMERIC-MANGO SMOOTHIE

Serves: *1*
Prep Time: *5*   Minutes

Cook Time: *5*   Minutes

Total Time: *10* Minutes

INGREDIENTS

- 1 cup Greek yogurt
- ¼ cup orange juice
- 1 banana
- 1 tablespoon turmeric
- 1 tsp vanilla extract
- 1 cup ice

DIRECTIONS

1. In a blender place all ingredients and blend until smooth
2. Pour smoothie in a glass and serve

AVOCADO-KALE SMOOTHIE

Serves: *1*

Prep Time: 5   Minutes

Cook Time: 5   Minutes

Total Time: *10*   Minutes

INGREDIENTS

- 1 cup coconut milk
- 1 tablespoon lemon juice
- 1 bunch kale
- 1 cup spinach
- ¼ avocado
- 1 cup ice

DIRECTIONS

1. In a blender place all ingredients and blend until smooth
2. Pour smoothie in a glass and serve

BUTTERMILK SMOOTHIE

Serves: *1*
Prep Time: 5   Minutes

Cook Time: 5   Minutes

Total Time: *10*   Minutes

INGREDIENTS

- 1 cup ice
- 1 cup strawberries
- 1 cup blueberries
- 1 cup buttermilk
- ½ tsp vanilla extract

DIRECTIONS

1. In a blender place all ingredients and blend until smooth
2. Pour smoothie in a glass and serve

Serves: **1**

Prep Time: **5** Minutes

Cook Time: **5** Minutes

Total Time: **10** Minutes

INGREDIENTS

- 1 cup berries
- 1 cup baby spinach
- 1 tablespoon orange juice
- ¼ cup coconut water
- ½ cup Greek yogurt

DIRECTIONS

1. In a blender place all ingredients and blend until smooth
2. Pour smoothie in a glass and serve

FRUIT SMOOTHIE

Serves: *1*
Prep Time: 5   Minutes

Cook Time: 5   Minutes

Total Time: *10* Minutes

INGREDIENTS

- 1 mango
- 1 cup vanilla yogurt
- 2 tablespoons honey
- 1 tablespoon lime juice
- 1 banana
- 1 can strawberries
- 1 kiwi

DIRECTIONS

1. In a blender place all ingredients and blend until smooth
2. Pour smoothie in a glass and serve

MANGO SMOOTHIE

Serves: *1*
Prep Time: *5*   Minutes

Cook Time: *5*   Minutes

Total Time: *10*   Minutes

INGREDIENTS

- 2 cups mango
- 1 cup buttermilk
- 1 tsp vanilla extract
- 1 cup kiwi
- ½ cup coconut milk

DIRECTIONS

1. In a blender place all ingredients and blend until smooth
2. Pour smoothie in a glass and serve

DREAMSICLE SMOOTHIE

Serves: **1**

Prep Time: **5**   Minutes

Cook Time: **5**   Minutes

Total Time: **10** Minutes

INGREDIENTS

- 1 cup Greek yogurt
- 1 cup ice
- ¼ cup mango
- 1 orange
- 1 pinch cinnamon

DIRECTIONS

1. In a blender place all ingredients and blend until smooth
2. Pour smoothie in a glass and serve

ICE-CREAM RECIPES

RICOTTA ICE-CREAM

Serves: *6-8*

Prep Time: *15*   Minutes

Cook Time: *15*   Minutes

Total Time: *30*   Minutes

INGREDIENTS

- 1 cup almonds
- 1-pint vanilla ice cream
- 2 cups ricotta cheese
- 1 cup honey

DIRECTIONS

1. In a saucepan whisk together all ingredients
2. Mix until bubbly
3. Strain into a bowl and cool
4. Whisk in favorite fruits and mix well
5. Cover and refrigerate for 2-3 hours
6. Pour mixture in the ice-cream maker and follow manufacturer instructions
7. Serve when ready

SAFFRON ICE-CREAM

Serves: *6-8*

Prep Time: *15*   Minutes
Cook Time: *15*   Minutes
Total Time: *30*   Minutes

INGREDIENTS

- 4 egg yolks
- 1 cup heavy cream
- 1 cup milk
- ½ cup brown sugar
- 1 tsp saffron
- 1 tsp vanilla extract

DIRECTIONS

1. In a saucepan whisk together all ingredients
2. Mix until bubbly
3. Strain into a bowl and cool
4. Whisk in favorite fruits and mix well
5. Cover and refrigerate for 2-3 hours
6. Pour mixture in the ice-cream maker and follow manufacturer instructions
7. Serve when ready

FOURTH COOKBOOK

SIDE DISHES

CAULIFLOWER STEAKS WITH LEMON SAUCE

Serves: **4**

Prep Time: **10** Minutes

Cook Time: **10** Minutes

Total Time: **20** Minutes

INGREDIENTS

- 1 head cauliflower
- 2 tablespoons olive oil
- 2 tsp paprika

LEMON SAUCE
- 1 cup parsley leaves
- ¼ cup mint leaves
- 1 garlic clove
- ¼ cup olive oil
- ¼ cup green onion
- Juice of 1 lemon

DIRECTIONS

1. In a blender add all ingredients for the lemon sauce and blend until smooth

2. For the cauliflower steak, cut cauliflower into thick slices and rub with olive oil

3. Sprinkle with spices and place the cauliflower in a skillet

4. Cook for 4-5 minutes per side

5. When ready remove and serve with lemon sauce

KUNG PAO CAULIFLOWER

Serves: **4**

Prep Time: **10**   Minutes

Cook Time: **30**   Minutes

Total Time: **40**   Minutes

INGREDIENTS

- 2 tablespoons olive oil
- salt
- 2 scallions
- ¼ cup cilantro
- 1 head cauliflower
- 1 tablespoon sesame seeds

SAUCE

- 1 tablespoon rice wine vinegar
- 1 tablespoon ginger
- 1 tsp olive oil
- 1 tablespoon soy sauce
- 1 tablespoon hoisin sauce

DIRECTIONS

1. In a bowl combine all sauce ingredients together and mix well

2. For the cauliflower heat the olive oil in a skillet and add the cauliflower

3. Add salt, sesame seeds and cook for 4-5 minutes

4. When ready remove from heat, add cilantro and stir to combine

5. Serve with sauce

RICE, KALE AND AVOCADO BOWL

Serves: 2

Prep Time: *10*   Minutes

Cook Time: *20*   Minutes

Total Time: *30*   Minutes

INGREDIENTS

- 1 cup rice
- 1 garlic clove
- 1 tablespoon rice vinegar
- 2 cups vegetable broth
- pinch of salt
- pinch of pepper
- 2 tablespoons
- 1 bunch kale
- 1 bunch kale
- 1 avocado

DIRECTIONS

1. In a pot stir in broth, rice and garlic
2. Bring to a simmer for and cook until liquid is evaporated
3. When ready toss rice with salt, pepper and vinegar
4. In another books toss kale with olive oil

5. Add kale and avocado slices to the rice
6. Serve when ready

CHICKEN MEATBALLS AND CAULIFLOWER RICE

Serves: **4**

Prep Time: **10**   Minutes

Cook Time: **30**   Minutes

Total Time: **40**   Minutes

INGREDIENTS

- ¼ cup red onion
- 1 lb. ground chicken
- 1 tablespoon mustard
- ¼ tsp black pepper
- 1 tablespoon olive oil
- 1 garlic clove
- ¼ cup parsley
- pinch of salt

SAUCE

- 1 cup parsley
- 1 can coconut milk
- 2 scallions
- zest of 1 lemon
- 1 cup ready-made cauliflower rice

DIRECTIONS

1. In a skillet heat olive oil and sauté onion and garlic for 3-4 minutes

2. Remove sautéed onion and garlic to a bowl

3. Stir in parsley, mustard, chicken, seasoning and mix well

4. Form balls from the mixture and place on a baking sheet

5. Bake at 400 F for 20 minutes

6. When ready remove from the oven and set aside

7. In a blender add all ingredients for the sauce and blend

8. Top the meatballs with sauce and cauliflower rice and serve

PINEAPPLE CHICKEN AND LETTUCE WRAPS

Serves: **2**

Prep Time: **10**   Minutes

Cook Time: **20**   Minutes

Total Time: **30**   Minutes

INGREDIENTS

- 2 cups cooked chicken
- 1 tablespoon olive oil
- ¼ tsp paprika
- 1 tablespoon lime juice
- ¼ tsp garlic powder
- ¼ tsp salt
- 1 cup pineapple cubes
- 8 lettuce wraps

DIRECTIONS

1. In a bowl combine garlic powder, lime juice, paprika, olive oil and lime juice
2. In your lettuce wraps add pineapple cubes, chicken and top with lime mixture
3. Serve when ready

ROASTED SALMON WITH POTATOES

Serves: **4**

Prep Time: **10**   Minutes

Cook Time: **35**   Minutes

Total Time: **45**   Minutes

INGREDIENTS

- 1 lb. potatoes
- 1 tsp lemon juice
- 4 salmon fillets
- ¼ tsp paprika
- 2 tablespoons olive oil

DIRECTIONS

1. Bake the potatoes at 375 F for 20-25 minutes
2. Rub the salmon fillets with paprika and olive oil
3. Bake the fish until golden brown
4. When ready from the oven and serve with baked potatoes and lemon juice

GUT ENERGY BOOSTING BOWL

Serves: *1*
Prep Time: 5   Minutes

Cook Time: 5   Minutes

Total Time: *10*   Minutes

INGREDIENTS

- 2 cups kale
- 1 tablespoon olive oil
- 1 avocado
- ¼ cup carrot
- ½ cup beans
- ¼ cup cabbage
- 1 cup baked potatoes

DIRECTIONS

1. In a bowl add all ingredients together
2. Drizzle olive oil and salt and mix well
3. Serve when ready

Serves: 2
Prep Time: 5   Minutes

Cook Time: 10   Minutes

Total Time: 15   Minutes

INGREDIENTS

- 2 zucchinis
- pinch of salt
- 2 avocados
- 2 tablespoons olive oil
- 2 eggs
- 1 tablespoon olive oil

DIRECTIONS

1. In a bowl toss the zucchini noodles with olive oil
2. Season and transfer to a baking sheet
3. Crack an egg over each portion
4. Bake for 8-10 minutes at 375 F
5. When ready remove from the oven and serve with avocado slices

CHICKEN WITH BAKED VEGGIES

Serves: **4**

Prep Time: **10**   Minutes

Cook Time: **30**   Minutes

Total Time: **40**   Minutes

INGREDIENTS

- 1 tablespoon olive oil
- 1 tablespoon honey
- 2 red bell peppers
- 2 carrots
- ¼ cup parsley
- 1 lb. chicken breast
- 2 onions

DIRECTIONS

1. Place the chicken onto a baking sheet
2. Add the rest of the ingredients to the chicken breast
3. Drizzle olive oil over chicken and veggies
4. Bake at 375 F for 25-30 minutes or until the vegetables are tender
5. When ready remove from the oven and serve

VEGGIE STIR-FRY

Serves: **2**

Prep Time: **10**   Minutes

Cook Time: **20**   Minutes

Total Time: **30**   Minutes

INGREDIENTS

- 1 tablespoon cornstarch
- 1 garlic clove
- ¼ cup olive oil
- ¼ head broccoli
- ¼ cup show peas
- ½ cup carrots
- ¼ cup green beans
- 1 tablespoon soy sauce
- ½ cup onion

DIRECTIONS

1. In a bowl combine garlic, olive oil, cornstarch and mix well
2. Add the rest of the ingredients and toss to coat
3. In a skillet cook vegetables mixture until tender
4. When ready transfer to a plate garnish with ginger and serve

GREEK PIZZA

Serves: **6-8**

Prep Time: **10** Minutes

Cook Time: **15** Minutes

Total Time: **25** Minutes

INGREDIENTS

- 1 pizza crust
- 1 tablespoon olive oil
- 6 oz. spinach
- ¼ cup basil
- 1 tsp oregano
- 1 cup mozzarella cheese
- 1 tomato
- ½ cup feta cheese

DIRECTIONS

1. Spread tomato sauce on the pizza crust
2. Place all the toppings on the pizza crust
3. Bake the pizza at 425 F for 12-15 minutes
4. When ready remove pizza from the oven and serve

Serves: **6-8**

Prep Time: **10** Minutes

Cook Time: **15** Minutes

Total Time: **25** Minutes

INGREDIENTS

- 1 cup cooked chicken breast
- ½ cup bbq sauce
- 1 pizza crust
- 1 tablespoon olive oil
- 1 cup cheese
- 1 cup tomatoes

DIRECTIONS

1. Spread tomato sauce on the pizza crust
2. Place all the toppings on the pizza crust
3. Bake the pizza at 425 F for 12-15 minutes
4. When ready remove pizza from the oven and serve

FIESTA SHRIMP

Serves: **1**
Prep Time: **5**   Minutes
Cook Time: **10** Minutes
Total Time: **15** Minutes

INGREDIENTS

- 3 oz. shrimp
- ¼ cup zucchini
- ½ cup fiesta garden salsa
- ¼ oz. cheese
- cilantro
- 1 tortilla

DIRECTIONS

1. In a bowl add zucchini, shrimp and pour salsa over
2. Microwave for 4-5 minutes and sprinkle with grated cheese and cilantro
3. Microwave tortilla for 10-20 seconds and serve with shrimp

CAULIFLOWER FRITTERS

Serves: *8*

Prep Time: *10*   Minutes

Cook Time: *30*   Minutes

Total Time: *40*   Minutes

INGREDIENTS

-   1 head of cauliflower
-   ¼ tsp chili powder
-   2 cloves garlic
-   2 tablespoons cilantro
-   1 tsp salt
-   ¼ tsp black pepper
-   2 eggs
-   3 tablespoons cornmeal
-   ½ cup flour
-   4 tablespoons nutritional yeast

DIRECTIONS

1. Cook cauliflower florets by steaming for 5-6 minutes
2. Mix the cauliflower with chili powder, cilantro, garlic, pepper and salt
3. In another bowl beat the egg, add cauliflower mixture, flour, cornmeal, and yeast

4. Add ¼ cup of the mixture to the pan and press down the fritter
5. Cook until golden brown for 3-4 minutes per side
6. When ready, remove and serve

Serves: 2
Prep Time: 5   Minutes

Cook Time: 10   Minutes

Total Time: 15   Minutes

INGREDIENTS

- 4 thin slices bread
- 2 eggs
- 1/3 cup almond milk
- ¼ tsp vanilla extract
- 1 tablespoon cream cheese
- 1 tablespoon apricot preserves
- ½ cup maple syrup

DIRECTIONS

1. In a bowl combine vanilla extract, eggs, almond milk, and mix well
2. Make 2 sandwiches with cream cheese and preserve
3. Place sandwiches in egg mixture on both sides
4. In a skillet cook sandwiches for 2-3 minutes per side or until golden brown
5. When ready remove and serve

GREEK MIXED VEGETABLES

Serves: **6**

Prep Time: **10**   Minutes

Cook Time: **90**   Minutes

Total Time: **100** Minutes

INGREDIENTS

- ½ cup olive oil
- 1 eggplant
- 1 onion
- 2 garlic cloves
- 1 lb. potatoes
- 5 tomatoes
- 10 cherry tomatoes
- 1 cup tomato passata
- 1 cup water
- 1 tablespoon dried oregano
- 1 tablespoon parsley
- 1 tsp salt

DIRECTIONS

1. Preheat the oven to 400 F
2. In a frying pan add olive oil, eggplant and cook for 6-7 minutes

3. Add garlic, onion and sauté for 5-6 minutes

4. Add potato, zucchini, passata, tomatoes, and water

5. Sprinkle with oregano, parsley, pepper, and salt

6. Mix well and transfer to a baking dish, drizzle with olive oil and bake for 45-55 minutes or until the top has browned

7. When ready remove and serve

GRILLED SALMON STEAKS

Serves: *4*

Prep Time: *5*   Minutes

Cook Time: *15*   Minutes

Total Time: *20*   Minutes

INGREDIENTS

- 2 salmon steaks
- 2 tablespoons dipping sauce
- 1 tsp cooking oil

DIRECTIONS

1. Heat grill and rub with cooking oil
2. Baste steaks with sauce
3. Cook for 4-5 minutes per side
4. Don't overcook
5. When ready remove and serve

ORIENTAL GREENS

Serves: *8*

Prep Time: *10*   Minutes

Cook Time: *90*   Minutes

Total Time: *100* Minutes

INGREDIENTS

- ¼ cup green beans
- ¼ cup snow peas
- 1 cup cauliflower florets
- 1 cup water chestnuts
- 2 radishes
- 2 scallions
- ½ cup red onion
- 1 tsp powdered ginger
- ½ cup rice wine vinegar

DIRECTIONS

1. In a bowl combine cauliflower floret, radish slices, onions, water chestnuts and mix well
2. In another bowl combine rice wine vinegar, powdered ginger and pour over vegetables
3. Refrigerate for 1-2 hours
4. When ready remove and serve

BROCCOLI CASSEROLE

Serves: **4**

Prep Time: **10** Minutes

Cook Time: **15** Minutes

Total Time: **25** Minutes

INGREDIENTS

- 1 onion
- 2 chicken breasts
- 2 tablespoons unsalted butter
- 2 eggs
- 2 cups cooked rice
- 2 cups cheese
- 1 cup parmesan cheese
- 2 cups cooked broccoli

DIRECTIONS

1. Sauté the veggies and set aside
2. Preheat the oven to 425 F
3. Transfer the sautéed veggies to a baking dish, add remaining ingredients to the baking dish
4. Mix well, add seasoning and place the dish in the oven
5. Bake for 12-15 minutes or until slightly brown
6. When ready remove from the oven and serve

RED ONION FRITATTA

Serves: *2*

Prep Time: *10*   Minutes

Cook Time: *20*   Minutes

Total Time: *30*   Minutes

INGREDIENTS

- ½ lb. asparagus
- 1 tablespoon olive oil
- ½ red onion
- ¼ tsp salt
- 2 eggs
- 2 oz. cheddar cheese
- 1 garlic clove
- ¼ tsp dill

DIRECTIONS

1. In a bowl whisk eggs with salt and cheese
2. In a frying pan heat olive oil and pour egg mixture
3. Add remaining ingredients and mix well
4. Serve when ready

SPINACH FRITATTA

Serves: **2**

Prep Time: **10**   Minutes

Cook Time: **20**   Minutes

Total Time: **30**   Minutes

INGREDIENTS

- ½ lb. spinach
- 1 tablespoon olive oil
- ½ red onion
- ¼ tsp salt
- 2 eggs
- 2 oz. cheddar cheese
- 1 garlic clove
- ¼ tsp dill

DIRECTIONS

1. In a bowl whisk eggs with salt and cheese
2. In a frying pan heat olive oil and pour egg mixture
3. Add remaining ingredients and mix well
4. Serve when ready

CHEESE FRITATTA

Serves: *2*

Prep Time: *10*   Minutes

Cook Time: *20*   Minutes

Total Time: *30*   Minutes

INGREDIENTS

- 1 tablespoon olive oil
- ½ red onion
- ¼ tsp salt
- 2 eggs
- 1 cup cheddar cheese
- 1 garlic clove
- ¼ tsp dill

DIRECTIONS

1. In a bowl whisk eggs with salt and cheese
2. In a frying pan heat olive oil and pour egg mixture
3. Add remaining ingredients and mix well
4. Serve when ready

RHUBARB FRITATTA

Serves: **2**

Prep Time: **10** Minutes

Cook Time: **20** Minutes

Total Time: **30** Minutes

INGREDIENTS

- 1 cup rhubarb
- 1 tablespoon olive oil
- ½ red onion
- ¼ tsp salt
- 2 oz. parmesan cheese
- 1 garlic clove
- ¼ tsp dill

DIRECTIONS

1. In a bowl whisk eggs with salt and parmesan cheese
2. In a frying pan heat olive oil and pour egg mixture
3. Add remaining ingredients and mix well
4. Serve when ready

BROCCOLI FRITATTA

Serves: *2*
Prep Time: *10*   Minutes

Cook Time: *20*   Minutes

Total Time: *30*   Minutes

INGREDIENTS

- 1 cup broccoli
- 1 tablespoon olive oil
- ½ red onion
- 2 eggs
- ¼ tsp salt
- 2 oz. cheddar cheese
- 1 garlic clove
- ¼ tsp dill

DIRECTIONS

1. In a bowl whisk eggs with salt and cheese
2. In a frying pan heat olive oil and pour egg mixture
3. Add remaining ingredients and mix well
4. Serve when ready

TOMATO RISOTTO

Serves: **2**

Prep Time: **10** Minutes

Cook Time: **25** Minutes

Total Time: **35** Minutes

INGREDIENTS

- 2-3 tablespoons olive oil
- 1 red onion
- 1 lb. vine-ripened tomatoes
- 1 lb. risotto rice
- 1 cup vegetable stock
- 1 cup cheese
- 2 oz. basil

DIRECTIONS

1. In a pan heat olive oil and sauté onion until soft
2. Place the tomatoes on a baking tray, drizzle olive oil and roast at 350 F for 18-20 minutes
3. Add the rice, stock to the pan and cook until rice is tender
4. Add the cheese, basil, tomatoes and serve when ready

Serves: **2**

Prep Time: **10**   Minutes

Cook Time: **50**   Minutes

Total Time: **60**   Minutes

INGREDIENTS

- 1 lb. butternut squash
- 3 tablespoons olive oil
- ¼ rolled pastry
- 2 eggs
- 200 ml double cream

DIRECTIONS

1. Roast the squash at 400 F for 18-20 minutes
2. Lay a baking paper on the pastry
3. Top with beans and bake for 12-15 minutes
4. Top the pastry with squash
5. Mix eggs, with double cream and pour over
6. Bake for another 20-25 minutes
7. When ready remove from the oven and serve

TOMATO TARTS

Serves: *2*
Prep Time: *10* Minutes

Cook Time: *35* Minutes

Total Time: *45* Minutes

INGREDIENTS

- 1 lb. pastry
- 2-3 tsp tomato paste
- 1 lb. tomatoes
- 1 tablespoons olive oil
- 1 tablespoon capers
- 1 lb. broccoli

DIRECTIONS

1. Unroll the pastry sheet and cut into rectangles
2. Spread tomato paste over each tart and drizzle olive oil
3. Scatter over capers
4. Bake at 400 F for 18-20 minutes
5. Meanwhile boil the broccoli for 12-15 minutes or until tender
6. When ready remove from the oven and serve with cooked broccoli

TOMATO AND ONION PASTA

Serves: *2*

Prep Time: *10*   Minutes

Cook Time: *20*   Minutes

Total Time: *30*   Minutes

INGREDIENTS

- 1 tablespoon olive oil
- 1 onion
- ½ lb. penne pasta
- 2-3 garlic cloves
- 1 oz. parsley
- ½ lb. tomatoes
- ¼ lb. low fat sour cream

DIRECTIONS

1. Heat olive oil in a pan and sauté onion until soft
2. Add pasta, garlic, pasta and water to cover
3. Bring to a boil and simmer for 5-6 minutes
4. Add tomatoes and cook for another 4-5 minutes
5. Drain the pasta mixture and return to the pan
6. Stir in soured cream
7. Garnish with parsley and serve

ROASTED SQUASH

Serves: **3-4**

Prep Time: **10**   Minutes

Cook Time: **20**   Minutes

Total Time: **30**   Minutes

INGREDIENTS

- 2 delicata squashes
- 2 tablespoons olive oil
- 1 tsp curry powder
- 1 tsp salt

DIRECTIONS

1. Preheat the oven to 400 F
2. Cut everything in half lengthwise
3. Toss everything with olive oil and place onto a prepared baking sheet
4. Roast for 18-20 minutes at 400 F or until golden brown
5. When ready remove from the oven and serve

Serves: *2*
Prep Time: *10*   Minutes

Cook Time: *20*   Minutes

Total Time: *30*   Minutes

INGREDIENTS

- 1 lb. brussels sprouts
- 1 tablespoon olive oil
- 1 tablespoon parmesan cheese
- 1 tsp garlic powder
- 1 tsp seasoning

DIRECTIONS

1. Preheat the oven to 425 F
2. In a bowl toss everything with olive oil and seasoning
3. Spread everything onto a prepared baking sheet
4. Bake for 8-10 minutes or until crisp
5. When ready remove from the oven and serve

PASTA

SIMPLE SPAGHETTI

Serves: 2

Prep Time: 5   Minutes

Cook Time: 15   Minutes

Total Time: 20   Minutes

INGREDIENTS

- 10 oz. spaghetti
- 2 eggs
- ½ cup parmesan cheese
- 1 tsp black pepper
- Olive oil
- 1 tsp parsley
- 2 cloves garlic

DIRECTIONS

1. In a pot boil spaghetti (or any other type of pasta), drain and set aside
2. In a bowl whish eggs with parmesan cheese
3. In a skillet heat olive oil, add garlic and cook for 1-2 minutes
4. Pour egg mixture and mix well
5. Add pasta and stir well

6. When ready garnish with parsley and serve

Serves: 2
Prep Time: 5   Minutes

Cook Time: 15   Minutes

Total Time: 20   Minutes

INGREDIENTS

- ¼ cup mayonnaise
- ¼ cup sweet chili sauce
- 1 tablespoon lime juice
- 1 garlic clove
- 8 z. pasta
- 1 lb. shrimp
- ¼ tsp paprika

DIRECTIONS

1. In a pot boil spaghetti (or any other type of pasta), drain and set aside
2. Place all the ingredients for the sauce in a pot and bring to a simmer
3. Add pasta and mix well
4. When ready garnish with parmesan cheese and serve

PASTA WITH OLIVES AND TOMATOES

Serves: **2**

Prep Time: **5**   Minutes

Cook Time: **15**   Minutes

Total Time: **20**   Minutes

INGREDIENTS

- 8 oz. pasta
- 3 tablespoons olive oil
- 2 cloves garlic
- 5-6 anchovy fillets
- 2 cups tomatoes
- 1 cup olives
- ½ cup basil leaves

DIRECTIONS

1. In a pot boil spaghetti (or any other type of pasta), drain and set aside
2. Place all the ingredients for the sauce in a pot and bring to a simmer
3. Add pasta and mix well
4. When ready garnish with parmesan cheese and serve

SALAD

TOMATO AND CUCUMBER SALAD

Serves: *1*

Prep Time: 5   Minutes

Cook Time: 5   Minutes

Total Time: *10*   Minutes

INGREDIENTS

- 2 cucumbers
- 2 tomatoes
- 2/3 cup red onion
- ½ cup balsamic vinegar
- ¼ tablespoons white vinegar
- 2 tablespoons olive oil
- basil leaves

DIRECTIONS

1. In a bowl combine all ingredients together and mix well
2. Serve with dressing

RADICCHIO AND TOMATO SALAD

Serves: *1*

Prep Time: *5*   Minutes

Cook Time: *5*   Minutes

Total Time: *10*   Minutes

INGREDIENTS

- 2 oz. radicchio
- 3 cups shredded romaine
- 8 cherry tomatoes
- 2 stalks celery
- 2 oz. cucumber
- 1 oz. garden cress
- 2 tsp olive oil
- 2 tsp vinegar

DIRECTIONS

1. In a bowl combine all ingredients together and mix well
2. Serve with dressing

BROCCOLI SALAD WITH CRANBERRIES

Serves: *1*

Prep Time: *5*   Minutes

Cook Time: *5*   Minutes

Total Time: *10*   Minutes

INGREDIENTS

- 3 cups broccoli florets
- ½ cup cranberries
- ½ cup sunflower seeds
- 2 apples
- ½ cup red onion
- 1 cup low-fat yoghurt
- ½ cup honey

DIRECTIONS

1. In a bowl combine all ingredients together and mix well
2. Serve with dressing

Serves: *1*
Prep Time: 5   Minutes

Cook Time: 5   Minutes

Total Time: *10*   Minutes

INGREDIENTS

- 1 head romaine lettuce
- 4 oz. smoked salmon
- 1 tomato
- 3 radishes
- 1 organic carrot
- ¼ cucumber
- 1 tsp ginger root
- 1 tablespoon canola oil

DIRECTIONS

1. In a bowl combine all ingredients together and mix well
2. Serve with dressing

SHRIMP AND EGGS SALAD

Serves: *1*
Prep Time: 5   Minutes

Cook Time: 5   Minutes

Total Time: *10*   Minutes

INGREDIENTS

- 2 cups shrimp
- ¼ cup cherry tomatoes
- ½ cup mayonnaise
- ½ cup chili sauce
- 2 tablespoons lemon juice
- romaine lettuce
- 2 hard-boiled eggs

DIRECTIONS

1. In a bowl combine all ingredients together and mix well
2. Serve with dressing

AVOCADO SALAD

Serves: **1**

Prep Time: **5**   Minutes

Cook Time: **5**   Minutes

Total Time: **10**   Minutes

INGREDIENTS

- 2 cups arugula leaves
- 2 cups cherry tomatoes
- ½ cup sun-dried tomatoes
- 2 tablespoons olive oil
- 1 tablespoon balsamic vinegar
- 1 avocado

DIRECTIONS

1. In a bowl combine all ingredients together and mix well
2. Serve with dressing

CHICKEN SALAD WITH PINE NUTS

Serves: **1**

Prep Time: **5**   Minutes

Cook Time: **5**   Minutes

Total Time: **10**   Minutes

INGREDIENTS

- 1 lb. chicken breast cooked
- ½ cup red onion
- ¼ cup cucumber
- ¼ cup basil
- ¼ cup cranberries
- 10 oz romaine lettuce

DRESSING

- 2 tablespoons balsamic vinegar
- 1 tablespoon canola oil
- 1 tablespoon honey
- 1 garlic clove
- salt
- black pepper
- ½ cup pine nuts

DIRECTIONS

1. In a bowl mix all ingredients and mix well
2. Serve with dressing

APPLE SALAD

Serves: *1*

Prep Time: 5   Minutes

Cook Time: 5   Minutes

Total Time: *10*   Minutes

INGREDIENTS

- 2 cups cooked chicken
- 1 cup grapes
- ¼ cup celery
- 2 tablespoons red onion
- ¼ cup apples
- 5 tablespoons mayonnaise
- 1 tsp lemon juice
- salt
- lettuce leaves

DIRECTIONS

1. In a bowl mix all ingredients and mix well
2. Serve with dressing

Serves: *1*
Prep Time: *5*   Minutes

Cook Time: *5*   Minutes

Total Time: *10*   Minutes

INGREDIENTS

- ½ cup raw beets
- ¼ cup carrots
- 1 tablespoon apple juice
- 1 tablespoon olive oil
- ½ tsp ginger
- ¼ tsp salt

DIRECTIONS

1. In a bowl combine all ingredients together and mix well
2. Serve with dressing

THANK YOU FOR READING THIS BOOK!

CPSIA information can be obtained
at www.ICGtesting.com
Printed in the USA
BVHW071211050421
604207BV00007B/728

9 781664 046092